PRAISE FOR
The Safe and Sane Guide to Teenage Plastic Surgery

"In an age where access to information about celebrities and teen idols undergoing plastic surgery to enhance their star qualities is virtually unlimited, the true benefits, as well as risks, of plastic surgery in teens is relatively scarce. Dr. Lukash, with examples culled from three decades of aesthetic and reconstructive surgery in teens, guides the potential teen patient and parent(s) through the details and necessary decisions required for both a safe and successful surgical outcome. This book's arrival could not be more timely and should remain a valuable resource for years to come."

—Bruce Bauer, MD
Director of Pediatric Plastic Surgery, Pritzker School of Medicine, University of Chicago; Coauthor of Principles of Pediatric Plastic Surgery; *Past President of the American Association of Pediatric Plastic Surgeons*

■ ■ ■

"I wish this book had existed when I was seventeen years old and facing reconstructive surgery. It would have been such a source of wisdom and comfort for not just me but for my parents, too. What a godsend this book will be for so many teens and their families."

—Jodee Blanco
New York Times *bestselling author of* Please Stop Laughing At Me...

■ ■ ■

"Great commonsense approach to the difficult image and perception problems that parents face during the teenage years of raising their children. No longer are we left to make these challenging and life-altering decisions on our own. Dr. Lukash's book reveals the how, when, and if plastic surgery can be beneficial in these formative years of development."

—Rod Rohrich, MD
Past President, American Society of Plastic Surgeons; Editor of the Journal of Plastic and Reconstructive Surgery; *and Chairman of the Department of Plastic Surgery, University of Texas Southwestern*

■ ■ ■

"At a time when the Internet and the media have influenced vulnerable young people in some worrisome ways, this book addresses the important clinical concerns about when plastic surgery may be an important consideration for young people and when it should be avoided. Often characterized as frivolous, plastic surgery can be critical for the well-being of a young person's psychological development. For the parent who is seriously contemplating plastic surgery for their teenager, Lukash provides an invaluable and up-to-date road map of when and how to proceed. Important issues to consider are outlined in a user-friendly fashion that will educate families about what it is that they need to be aware of. Comprehensive and easy to read, this resource will educate those contemplating plastic surgery and answer many of the important questions that they may have. This is an important reference on the topic of plastic surgery for teens."

—Victor Fornari, MD
Director of Child and Adolescent Psychiatry, North Shore University Hospital & Long Island Jewish Medical Center; Professor of Psychiatry, Hofstra University School of Medicine

■ ■ ■

"I felt as though I was talking to a very well-educated friend, as the book did not 'speak down' to me or make any of my concerns seem unjustified. It made the parents' as well as the child's feelings heard and addressed."

—Donna Halperin
Editor-in-Chief and CEO of Long Island Image Magazine

The
Safe and **Sane**
Guide to
TEENAGE
PLASTIC
SURGERY

The
Safe and Sane
Guide to
TEENAGE
PLASTIC
SURGERY

FREDERICK N. LUKASH, MD
FACS, FAAP

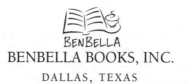

BenBELLA
BENBELLA BOOKS, INC.
DALLAS, TEXAS

BenBella Books, Inc.
10300 N. Central Expressway, Suite 400
Dallas, TX 75231
www.benbellabooks.com
Send feedback to feedback@benbellabooks.com

Printed in the United States of America
10 9 8 7 6 5 4 3 2 1

Library of Congress Cataloging-in-Publication Data is available for this title.
978-1-935618-09-6

Editing by Debbie Harmsen
Copyediting by Rebecca Green
Proofreading by Kyle Avery
Cover design by Faceout
Text design and composition by John Reinhardt Book Design
Procedure illustrations by Paige Jackson
Printed by Bang Printing

Distributed by Perseus Distribution
(www.perseusdistribution.com)

To place orders through Perseus Distribution:
Tel: 800-343-4499
Fax: 800-351-5073
E-mail: orderentry@perseusbooks.com

Significant discounts for bulk sales are available.
Please contact Glenn Yeffeth at glenn@benbellabooks.com or (214) 750-3628.

This book is dedicated to the memory of two individuals
who have been strong influences in my life both personally
and professionally:

Leslie Lukash, MD (1920–2007),
Chief Medical Examiner of Nassau County and my father,
a role model and moral compass.

I wish he could have read this book.

And to

Robert Goldwyn, MD (1930–2010),
plastic surgeon, teacher, mentor, and friend.

I am glad he was able to read the book.

Acknowledgments

The making of a book like this entails the dedicated work of many people.

First and foremost, I would like to thank my patients, without whom you would not be holding this book in your hands. Their stories have inspired and directed my path as a physician since I first began my practice.

Second, I must thank my wife, Yaffa, and my children, Sarah, Abigail, and Molly, for their unflagging support through the process, which often meant letting me go off into my study and write throughout a long, busy year.

To my agent, Katharine Sands of the Sarah Jane Freymann Literary Agency; my collaborative writer, Gretchen Kelly; my publisher, BenBella; and to my editor, Debbie Harmsen. Thank you for saying "yes" and for helping make this long-held dream a reality.

To Marc Gerstein, PhD, and Robert Berg, DMD, a special thanks for your encouraging yet critical input.

To Glenn Pollack, PhD; Howard Green, MD; and Victor Fornari, MD, for your invaluable insight into the psychological world of school-age children.

To Deborah Sarnoff, MD, and Jeanette Graff, MD, for your help with information about nonsurgical dermatology.

To Robert M. Goldwyn, MD, my mentor and friend, for always believing this project was important.

To Bruce Bauer, MD, for taking time to review and critique this manuscript.

With heartfelt thanks, I would also like to acknowledge those children whose emotional artistic expressions gathered over more than thirty years served as the genesis for this book. Some of them appeared in my landmark article "Children's Art as an Index of Self Esteem in Plastic Surgery" (*Journal of Plastic and Reconstructive Surgery* May 2002) and are included in this book.

I am also grateful for the many letters and attestations from patients and parents confirming the benefits of quality-of-life surgery when appropriate. For privacy concerns their names have been changed; but the message has not.

Thank you, too, to those teens and adolescents, and their parents, for consenting inclusion of their before and after photographs. Plastic surgery is a visual specialty and images can surpass words in telling the story.

And last, thank you to my readers for trusting me with your healing, your hopes, and your dreams. We have started this journey together. My very best for your ongoing quest for the best in life.

Contents at a Glance

Complete Table of Contents

PART TWO
PROCEDURES

PART THREE
POSTSURGERY

Introduction

I N 2009, close to 300,000 teens underwent aesthetic plastic surgery.
Those numbers are rising. And for every teen who underwent
plastic surgery, ten more are online right now researching the procedure they've been thinking about during each gym session, sleepover
party, and school dance. Most of these teens aren't dreaming about looking like Barbie or Ken or even Rihanna, Beyoncé, Gwyneth, or Justin.
They're just longing to fit in, to look like everyone else.

Your son or daughter might be among them.

As a plastic surgeon with thirty years of successful practice, I know
for sure that fitting in physically *does* matter. It is why we shower, brush
our teeth, comb our hair, and carefully choose our wardrobe. It is why
gyms are crowded and the diet industry is booming.

How we look is linked intimately to how we feel. And the emotions
related to how we look and feel are not dictated by age. Just because you
are young does not mean that you feel great about your appearance—or
that you feel, as the French so aptly put it, *bien dans sa peau*—"well in
one's skin."

While adults are most often seeking rejuvenating (a.k.a. "fountain
of youth") procedures, teens aren't looking to stand out; they just want
to feel "normal." Existing under the bell curve of average is what they
want. Anything out of the norm—breasts that are too big or too small,
ears that stick out, noses that dominate their faces—wreaks havoc on

1

their emotions. When teens fit in, looks become the background to the rest of their living. When they don't fit in, their appearance and how they feel about it becomes all consuming.

Take the example of Tom, age 15, who suffered from the physical and psychological stress of having male "breasts," an embarrassing condition called gynecomastia that is often caused by an imbalance of hormones. Here is what he wrote to me:

> I want to share my feelings about my "breasts." I wasn't confident at all. I felt that people were staring at me. All I would wear was black to hide this "horrible defect." When I found out that something could be done, I was very excited. My doctor made me feel comfortable about what I had and how it could be fixed.
>
> The surgery was easy, and the recovery time at home was a mere week.
>
> I was incredibly pleased with the results. I can barely see any scarring. Now I wear any color I want and am much more confident. I can go around not feeling like everyone is staring at me. I can live my life!
> —Tom (former patient)

Or take this example from my teenage patient Sophie:

> In my earlier years, all I wanted was to fit in with the "in" crowd. At the time, I felt that there was only one thing stopping me—that thing being my big nose. Kids made fun of me and called me names. I was the small kid with the big nose: not how you want to be identified.
>
> As early as sixth grade the social pain was unbearable. My mother took me to a plastic surgeon who specializes in children. Even though a surgery would be limited and the result might change as I grew, I needed it.
>
> Once I had the surgery I felt more in balance. I made many friends, and not the ones in the "in" crowd—good friends who liked me for who I am. The procedure helped bring out the best in me.
> —Sophie (former patient)

My specialty is pediatric plastic surgery. That means that I am considered an expert in working with youngsters who are in a critical stage of development, both mentally and physically, and that I am trained to structurally (that is, physically) make people feel whole. Through reconstructive plastic surgery, I establish (or reestablish, as the case may be) a quality of life robbed by an accident of birth, trauma, or disease. I cannot remake people, but I can refine and balance parts that are out of alignment with the norms of attractiveness. Plastic surgery is a way to do that, and it yields results that are more than physical changes. Teens who feel confident about their appearance are more apt to do better in school, form more cohesive social bonds, and build the foundations of psychological wellness that will last a lifetime.

Plastic comes from the Greek *plastikos*—"to shape or mold." Plastic surgery, therefore, is one specialty that reshapes or reestablishes structure. Over time it has come to mean different things to different people. For those with deformities, it is the hope for normalcy. For others, including many baby boomers, it is a way to re-create a more youthful or sexy look. Between the purely reconstructive and the purely cosmetic are the shades of gray where plastic surgery can be quality-of-life surgery. And that is how I see it for teenagers. To drive home my point, let me say that again: **At its best, teen plastic surgery is quality-of-life surgery.**

Young people are subjected to many stresses in their fast-paced lives. One of the biggest stressors for them is the need for acceptance by their peers. Those with aesthetic issues can become severely disillusioned with themselves and actually fail to thrive. Where do we draw the line for who deserves quality-of-life correction? Who determines what is a true deformity and what is only perceived to be one? Is it the teen, the parent, the doctor? Do we need a psychiatrist? Should the teen just rise above the feelings and learn to live with the cards he has been dealt? Or should skill and technology help people achieve a balance and harmony and greater happiness within?

If you are holding this book in your hands right now, I believe that you agree with me that improving a teen's life by structurally improving his or her physical appearance to conform to normal standards of attractiveness is a good thing. I'm not talking about breast enhancements before age 18 or about creating Michael Jackson-like clones. My hair curls on end when I see programs like *Dr. 90210*, *Extreme Makeover*, *The Swan*, *Miami Slice*, and even *Nip/Tuck*. I did not enter into medicine and plastic surgery to watch it become trivialized and sensationalized. I am an in-the-trenches doctor, trying to improve the lives of my patients through structural surgery. I want to make a life-altering positive impact on those who feel uncomfortable in their own skins.

This book is important because it brings relevance to a teen's feelings about his or her appearance in our high-pressure society. I wrote it not for self-promotion but to help people understand the difference between lasting beneficial changes and quick fixes (in other words, what some teens may see as an "easy out" to their problems). I wrote it to let parents know that there are ethical surgeons out there who do care about their work, who will say "no" as well as "yes." If a teen chooses surgery, it needs to be the right procedure for the right reason at the right time.

The power of plastic surgery to restore self-esteem, self-confidence, and self-empowerment to kids is incredible. This is not what most people think about when they think of plastic surgery. Yet I have seen the miracle of healing a child who feels diminished and powerless because of physical attributes outside the norm. Again, we are not talking about vanity here; we are talking about feeling normal.

I have received hundreds of heartfelt letters and emails from my patients and their parents postsurgery. This is from the mother of Mitchell, a teen whose "jug" ears had made his life a misery:

> This letter comes with [our] sincerest gratitude for the incredible positive changes in our lives since Mitchell's otoplasty.
>
> Before surgery Mitchell was ridiculed beyond belief. His life was consumed with quick comebacks from derisive comments. Fun with kids his own age was foreign. He was often alone during recess and his grades suffered.
>
> Mitchell is now a well-adjusted, popular, and well-liked young man. He is very sociable and fashionable. He likes girls and is liked in return. His world has opened up. He now excels academically.
>
> Gone are the endless tears. Now the only tears are those of

joy. we will always be grateful for the care our doctor took to change not only our little boy's life but the lives of those around him.

—Roseann (mother of teenage boy)

About Me

The focus of my practice has been pediatric plastic surgery, the care of structural issues for children under 22. My dedication to children began early in my education. In 1965, during my first week of school at Tulane University, the city of New Orleans was dealing with the aftermath of Hurricane Betsy. I spent that time volunteering to help clean up the city. I aided in the cleanup efforts by repairing and repainting an orphanage. Decades later during Hurricane Katrina, I helped to raise $40,000 for the Newcomb College Nursery School.

Throughout my career I have volunteered my skills, doing pro bono work for kids who have had physical defects but cannot afford traditional plastic surgery.

In 1986, I went to Guatemala with Surgical Aid to Children of the World and operated and lectured. I brought back a teenager with lye injuries and repaired her defects. A year later I volunteered to treat Afghan children who were disfigured during the war with the Russians. I have worked pro bono off and on over the years for Little Flower Children and Family Services to help correct children's disfigurements so that they have a better chance for placement and adoption. This past year, I operated on a brother and sister in Puerto Rico who had a cleft lip and palate.

For thirty years I have helped children be their best physically. I have experienced my patients' joys and sorrows, and I have witnessed surgical improvements that have so elevated their spirits that anything becomes possible for them. I have documentation for some of these transformations thanks to the many written testimonies of teens and parents I've received over the years. I include many of these attestations in the pages of this book. I also include some artwork from my patients to illustrate how rejected they feel when they don't fit in with their peers and then how wonderful they feel after their plastic surgeries. The results affirm to me the positive impact that surgery for the right child at the right time can have.

As the father of three daughters, I have the perspective of not only a doctor but also a parent wanting to see my children happy and thriving. I have watched them grow and seen their successes and failures as well as their frustrations, including dissatisfaction with their looks. One daughter requested nothing from me as a plastic surgeon; the other two desired nose surgeries, which my wife and I considered with each daughter individually (see chapter 8 for details).

Why This Book?

In my three decades of studying the effects of body image on the self-esteem of children and teens, I have amassed a body of knowledge that I want to pass on to others. This book is a guide for parents and their sons and daughters through the wilderness of teen angst, body image, and self-esteem. It is not a frivolous manual on how to be beautiful. It does not propose to equate beauty with success. It *does* discuss the value society places on appearance and the impact that societal pressure has on teens. This book aims to be of service to children with structural-appearance issues. I sincerely believe that there are many teens and their families out there who need practical, factual, and compassionate advice on the very real benefits of corrective plastic surgery.

The idea for this book is decades old. It began with the art I collected from children regarding their feelings about their looks and continued through the follow-up testaments, from which I learned of the positive impact I've had on individual lives. It would have been easy to simply surrender to the daily grind of practice and avoid the extra effort required to make this book happen. Many times I thought of doing just that, but the smile on the face of a child I'd helped would bring me back to the reality that this book needed to be written.

The project was not easy. Public opinion is, to say the least, polarized on such a hot-button subject. Many publishing houses rejected this book, calling it "too controversial."

I was about to throw in the towel when I showed part of the book to a public relations firm. The owner/agent looked at the work and said that she had never seen a surgeon so dedicated to the well-being of adolescents. She could not believe that there was such a passionate advocate for pediatric plastic surgery. When I showed her the letters from patients I operated on years ago, she was astounded that I follow "my kids" throughout their adolescence into adulthood. When she asked why, I stated the obvious—I wanted to know how their lives turned out and that I'd made a positive difference. Helping these young people, not money or fame, is what transcends everything I do. I have been to confirmations, bar and bat mitzvahs, and even weddings of the kids I have treated. I have become part of their families. Parents call me for advice because they know I care about their kids. I become emotional when a grandparent tells me that he thinks of me every day because of what I did for his loved one.

I want parents to gain a sense of trust in the benefits of plastic surgery when they read this book. There are real answers to real problems. Adolescents have feelings that need to be addressed and we need to listen to them.

When I wrote the book and could not get a publisher, many agents actually wanted it to be even more controversial—give the audience something sensational about kids and cosmetic surgery, they said. I could not do it. Too much emotion goes into my daily life in dealing with kids with great sorrow and angst to pander to the "Barbie Goes for Plastic Surgery" angle.

I wrote the position paper on teenage plastic surgery for the American Society of Plastic Surgeons (ASPS). I served on the public education committee for ASPS, trying to get sensible messages about plastic surgery out to the public. I've spent many hours battling the public perception that kids are just too young to know their own feelings. My experience told me otherwise. This book is the compilation of all those efforts. Kudos to BenBella Books, which also saw the need for this important guide.

What This Book Will Do for You

This book will assist you in deciding whether or not plastic surgery solutions are right for your child. It will illustrate when "no" is the right answer and when "yes" should at least be considered. It will give you understanding of the emotional turmoil your son or daughter may feel in regard to his or her appearance. It offers practical advice from professional health care providers and notes the signals to look for when body image is affecting self-esteem. Insight from psychologists and psychiatrists is complemented by real-life stories from young people who've dealt with negative body-image issues. This book will guide you to the right sources for help.

Teens have voices that need to be heard. They can, with their parents, come to realistic decisions about appearance and surgery. Plastic surgery isn't always the answer, but when it is, it can be safe, sane, and successful.

Not only parents will find this book useful. Psychologists, social workers, child psychiatrists, pediatricians, and others who work with young people will be able to use it to add to their knowledge on the subject. Plastic surgeons who only occasionally treat teens can use the book to gain insight into dealing with this special subset of patients and families.

Above all, the book is meant to be of service—to put the vast and life-affirming benefits of plastic surgery into the hands of those who need them.

How to Work with This Book

The book can be read in its entirety, or it can be used as a reference for specific problems. Part 1 addresses body image and self-esteem and how to start a dialogue with your teens about what they're feeling. It also discusses the cost and how to decide if surgery is the solution. It isn't always the answer. There are red flags that serve as warnings against surgery, such as body dysmorphic disorder (BDD), as well as green lights that help you know when to go forward with surgery. There are also flashing lights that help you proceed with caution when another discipline—such as psychiatry—is involved.

Part 2 covers the types of surgeries available and what to expect from each in terms of the surgical procedure, realistic results, and recovery. Part 3 looks at the plastic surgery industry as a whole—past, present, and future.

PART ONE

DECIDING IF PLASTIC SURGERY IS RIGHT FOR YOUR TEEN

1

Body Image

"Watching your child suffer is the hardest burden a parent can have. Kristin had only one breast that developed. No cover-up could make her look normal. Her sense of self was so compromised that she would not go out and socialize and in fact developed ulcers over the anxiety of not fitting in. There was no consoling her, and psychological counseling only made her feel worse. This was a cruel burden to place on a young soul."

"Buckets of tears were shed each day as I watched my child try and battle the day outside the comfort of our home. Mitchell had what his so-called friends referred to 'monkey' ears and 'Dumbo the elephant' ears. He could not keep up emotionally, and his socialization and grades plummeted. The expression 'kids can be cruel' was so true."

THESE ARE THE KINDS OF STORIES I hear from parents. Living like this is a reality many teens face. "Jughead," "Parrot Beak," "Hooter Girl," and "Girly Man" are just some of the epithets some teens endure when a body part is structurally different. This name-calling can make the ridiculed body part difficult to adjust to. The physical attribute that bothers each of these teens may be different, but the isolation, the feelings of inferiority, and the teasing from classmates haunt them just the same.

Perceptions versus Reality

Your teen lives in a world where judgments are made superficially and subjectively—sometimes even arbitrarily. Society has placed a value on good looks and rewards those who have them. Every day your child receives messages and signals about appearance, and not just when he or she is in school. What society considers attractive comes through in overt and subliminal ways—dialogue in sitcoms, billboard advertisements, videos on MTV and YouTube, discussions online, fashion spreads in *Teen Vogue*, and so on. A recent study cited in *Teen Decisions: Body Image* (Ojeda 2002) showed that by the time a girl reaches age 17, she has been exposed to more than 250,000 media bytes on beauty.

And every media personality, it seems, is beautiful. To a teen, attractiveness equals success.

In Nancy Etcoff's book *Survival of the Prettiest: The Science of Beauty* (1999), she writes that many intellectuals argue that beauty is inconsequential. They say, "It explains nothing, teaches nothing, and solves nothing." Etcoff notes, however, that outside this theoretical realm, beauty and appearance do rule.

In other words, what may be *rationally* correct is not necessarily *emotionally* correct. Appearance matters!

How someone looks affects how he or she is treated. One preschool study, "Physical Attractiveness and Peer Perception Among Children" (Dion and Berscheid 1974), showed that teachers and staff gave more attention to the more attractive children and were more tolerant with them for transgressions than they were with those they found less attractive. The adults presumed the more attractive children to be more intelligent as well.

Steve Jeffes, author of *Appearance Is Everything* (1998), relates similar findings. He says attractive people are assumed to be smart, capable, personable, and better at the art of persuasion than less attractive people—and that this appearance discrimination occurs at every age. Because of people's presumptions, those who are deemed attractive tend to be treated better and are more socially accepted. This is especially hard on children, because the way they are treated by parents, teachers, coaches, other adults, and peers contributes to their inner development.

In my thirty years of treating children and adolescents as a plastic surgeon, I have spent a significant amount of time researching the psychological aspects of body image. There are well-documented relationships between negative body image and low self-esteem. And even though a healthy view of self has many components—intelligence, effort, talent, appearance—these components are not always equal, and in various situations, one component may supersede another.

In reality, we know that looks do not constitute a person's worth. Unfortunately, a common perception is that they might. Placing value on attractiveness is hardwired into our biology. Attractiveness signals health and vitality, and those who possess it are at a social advantage. It is also true that the perception can become the reality. If your teen feels bad about his or her body, there may be spin-off into other aspects of life.

Children and teens are by nature social creatures. They are extremely observant and are quick to notice if someone is being treated better than they are. They pick up on this preferential treatment not just by other kids but by adults as well—who is the teacher's pet, for example. In school and community activities, kids see peer groups forming and cliques being established. They rapidly learn that like attracts like and tends to stay away from those who are dissimilar. (This happens in adulthood, too, with fraternities and sororities, country clubs, and other exclusive groups.)

Those who are deemed attractive tend to be treated better and are more socially accepted. This is especially hard on children, because the way they are treated by parents, teachers, coaches, other adults, and peers contributes to their inner development.

Our sense of self begins early in life. Praise reinforces, and criticism is destructive to the developing ego. A child's early confidence translates into long-term emotional strength. This is why it's important to discuss body-image issues with your child early on if you believe her view of herself physically is affecting her self-esteem.

As a summer camp counselor and as a high school fencing coach, I witnessed those who succeeded and those who struggled. Some succeeded on their looks, others on their athleticism, and still others on their brains. Others failed on some, or all, levels. They were either part of the crowd or separate from the crowd—and that made all the difference in their self-esteem.

As a physician and pediatric plastic surgeon, I have felt the sadness and the angst of families whose lives have been challenged by something completely beyond their control. I have seen children at a fork in the road of their lives: They could alter their appearances through surgery or they could continue to endure taunting and teasing so disruptive that they chose to limit themselves physically to the sanctuary of home.

You, as a parent, may be wondering how to tell if your teen is suffering or struggling with body-image issues. The earliest of signs are usually behavioral. I call these "nonverbal" cues. Teens who have a negative body image can act in unpredictable ways. Some might simply seek anonymity and try to blend in. Others may act out to divert attention from their physical features; this could be seen in scenarios such as getting tattoos, letting their grades slip, or picking on other kids. Or they'll shut down and turn inward to avoid communication.

Altered behavior is not always a result of body-image issues, but it may be—especially if your teen perceives he or she has a physical flaw. If the behavior has started recently, it could be that something or someone has triggered negative feelings in your teen about his or her appearance. It might have been a derisive comment or a comparison to another individual. If you suspect that your teen may be acting out because of a body issue, do not be afraid to question individuals who are involved with your teen: teachers, coaches, camp counselors. If there is a change in his or her social behavior, speak to your child's friends. You may think this is an invasion of his or her privacy, but it may illuminate the situation, providing you valuable information so you can help your child.

Sir William Osler, MD, a world-famous physician in the 1900s, commented, "Listen to your patient. He is trying to tell you what is wrong." These words are applicable to parents and all who are concerned with a teen's welfare. Often, the way a teen will "tell" you that something is wrong is not through words but through actions.

I once had a teen patient whose parents first realized there was a problem when he suddenly refused to take a shower after gym class. He was sent to the principal's office, where nothing was resolved. A short time later, the class was playing basketball in a "shirts vs. skins" game.

Nonverbal Cues That Your Teen May Have Body-image Issues

- Refuses to go shopping
- Refuses to go to camp
- Refuses to go to the beach
- Refuses to engage socially (e.g., won't go to school functions, be involved in clubs, or participate on teams)
- Acts out in school (e.g., becomes "class clown," "class bully," or "class dummy")
- Begins to dress differently (e.g., wearing all black or loose cover-up clothing)
- Changes hairstyles or keeps his head slouched to cover up features he is unhappy about, such as his ears or nose
- Changes eating and exercise habits in an attempt to lose weight in some area (e.g., to make breasts smaller)
- Avoids conversations about appearance or fails to communicate in general
- Attempts to take control of her body with defiant acts (e.g., piercings, tattoos)
- Becomes resentful and jealous of others who have what she wants
- Becomes frustrated over any situation that he cannot control
- Starts doing poorly in classes

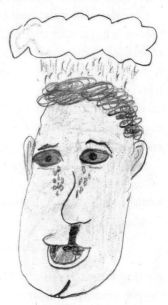

A 12-year-old boy depicts a vivid awareness that he is different from his peers. In his drawing, he illustrates his "problem," letting us know of his unhappiness with both tears and clouds of rain.

He refused to take his shirt off. He became verbally abusive to the teacher when a power struggle ensued. He was again in the principal's office, but he was closemouthed about the issue. His parents also noticed he was no longer going to the beach with his friends. His pediatrician had observed some abnormal breast development, but because the teen had not vocalized any concern, he'd put off the issue for a future follow-up. There were many signs that could have led to a discussion and early resolution. Once the parents finally eased into a discussion with their son about the issue, which brought it out into the open, the teen was overjoyed to learn that something could be done.

One sign that a girl may be having body-image issues with overly large breasts is aggressive dieting. Sometimes teens who are overdeveloped but otherwise of normal weight will start starvation diets, thinking they will reduce their breast size. They may have been influenced by pictures of celebrities who, through their sensationalized diets, have reduced their size and breasts. Although weight loss in overweight girls will result in a reduction of breast mass, if your teen is already of normal weight, dieting is an unhealthy and ultimately unsuccessful way to try to resolve the issue.

It is crucial for parents to understand that while teens don't always talk about their situations, they may be trying to communicate a problem through their actions, feelings, and responses.

Talking with Your Teen

Getting your teen to talk about a problem may be difficult. She may be deeply embarrassed or may be unaware of some of her own feelings about her body. Sometimes the topic, even tactfully brought up, will cause anger, humiliation, and tears. But it is your duty as the parent to begin the conversation.

Starting a dialogue is the most difficult step. Anyone with experience with teens knows how tricky this can be on almost any subject. Teens tend to speak and respond on their own terms. If you have picked up a cue that your teen has a problem with self-esteem and body image, you cannot just broach the topic without the potential of emotional backlash. It would be wonderful if a parent could just confront the issue and work to resolve it, but with teens, this is not always so easy and parents should generally approach the subject more delicately. This is especially true when there are multiple issues to contend with—some that can be resolved by behavior modification and others that are beyond an individual's control because of they way his or her body is structured.

A behavioral therapist can help you and your child understand behavioral issues. You may start by consulting your pediatrician, describing the cues you have seen, and asking for a recommendation. If the issues are at school, a school psychologist or social counselor may have recommendations that can help you open up a dialogue.

Psychologists are skilled at interpreting both verbal and nonverbal signals that a body-image issue may be at fault for behavioral problems. They can assess postures, gestures, rumblings, and voice changes as well as silence. Unlike parents, these professionals are in a position to offer an objective viewpoint and a neutral setting, which may allow a teen to feel more comfortable talking to them. By fitting the pieces together and gaining your teen's trust, they can get your teen to start talking and reveal the emotional impact of the physical issue. Psychologists can speak compassionately and supportively to a distressed teen and then professionally communicate with his pediatrician for more insight without violating the teen's sense of privacy.

> Psychologists are skilled at interpreting both verbal and nonverbal signals that a body-image issue may be at fault for behavioral problems. They can assess postures, gestures, rumblings, and voice changes as well as silence.

Once a psychologist has built a bond of trust with a teen, he or she can begin a conversation about treatment options. This opens the door for parents to ease into the discussion without their teen perceiving them as adversarial.

Dr. Glenn Pollack, head of the psychology department at State University of New York at Purchase, where he works with children as they transition into adulthood, says it is the role of parents to initiate conversation about a teen's body-image concerns.

"Many teens feel self-conscious and reluctant to discuss personal issues relating to body image," he says. "They may be experiencing feelings of guilt or embarrassment and find it difficult to initiate a conversation. So, your role as parent is to initiate conversation."

He gives the following tips for how to initiate and maintain a fruitful discussion:

- **Observe.**
  Watch for signs of distress. Pick up on cues—verbal and nonverbal. You know when your teen is not acting like himself, so go with your gut!

- **Don't Be Afraid.**
  Initiating a conversation about an area of concern with your son or daughter won't make the problem worse.
- **Show Empathy and Be Nonjudgmental.**
  As a parent you have strong beliefs, but this is about having a back-and-forth discussion, not trying to prove that you are right. Your teen will sense if you really want to discuss and listen rather than simply give orders.
- **Understand.**
  Synthesize and rephrase what your teen is expressing so that she knows you "get" what she is really saying and feeling. Help her to continue the dialogue.
- **Plan the Timing—But Be Flexible.**
  Be prepared at any time to have this discussion, because you never know when your teen might open up. However, if you're planning to start the conversation, choose an appropriate time—not when your teen is preoccupied.
- **Clarify Thoughts and Feelings.**
  Help your teen identify his thoughts, emotions, and behaviors. Keep your questions open-ended rather than asking ones that need only a yes-or-no response. For example, ask, "Can you let me know more about it?"
- **Don't Fix It.**
  Parents desperately want to eliminate their child's emotional distress. As a result, they can minimize the child's feelings. For example, a parent might say, "Don't worry, you look fine." Or, "You shouldn't feel that way." Don't do this. Having a dialogue is about letting your teen express himself freely and about listening and understanding his thoughts and feelings.
- **Know Your Limits.**
  Although you probably know more than your son or daughter about his or her area of concern, encourage further investigation of the issue. You can work as a team in gathering additional information to come up with a solution.
- **Remember: Rome Wasn't Built in a Day.**
  You don't have to discuss and solve everything in one conversation. Establishing an atmosphere of understanding and

respect will encourage your child to have additional discussions with you.

- **Back Away If It's Too Hot to Handle.**
  If the discussion becomes heated, cool it off with some downtime. You can resume the conversation later.
- **Don't Personalize.**
  This is not about you; it's about the emotional distress your teenager is experiencing. Becoming defensive will only shut down a dialogue.
- **Don't Mind Read.**
  Don't assume you know what your teen is thinking and feeling. Encourage her to disclose her thoughts to you rather than tell her what she is thinking or feeling.
- **Don't Try to Be a Fortune-Teller.**
  All too often parents get caught up with how terrible things will turn out in the future if a "wrong" decision is even talked about. Discussing the issue at hand in the present will enhance the dialogue.
- **Exercise Your Positive Parental Power.**
  Although they are on a journey toward autonomy, teens still need your praise, hugs, smiles, and other encouragement. Your job is to empower them to paddle through the rapids—but you can calm the waters sometimes, too.

2

Considering
Plastic Surgery

I F EVER THERE WAS a hot-button issue, teenage plastic surgery is
it. Advocates feel it can have the positive effect of healing the mind
as much as the body. Adversaries denigrate it as an easy way out or
a product of mere vanity; and they are usually the ones who need it the
least.

Those who argue against surgical correction in young people for the
sake of body image and self-esteem are often transferring adult reasons
for surgery onto children. Children are not small adults! As I mentioned
previously, adults who choose plastic surgery are often searching for
that fountain of youth or sexier look, but teens are simply looking to
fit in.

As a society, we are comfortable with and relieved that there are surgeons who can treat those deformed by birth, trauma, or disease. It
gives us hope that if one of our own were afflicted, there would be help
for him or her. Conversely, we are uncomfortable with—yet intrigued
by—celebrities and wannabes who subject themselves to extreme procedures on a whim. Somewhere in between are real teens who are not
truly deformed but also not driven by narcissism.

Whether a teen is suffering because of peer pressure, media-imposed standards of beauty, or a self-realization that he or she is uncomfortably different, the effect is the same: Personality and behavior can be severely altered when a young person feels awkward in his own skin.

How Surgery Can Boost Self-esteem

If you started this book by reading the introduction, you know a good deal about me and how my lifelong passion has been pediatric plastic surgery and its impact on body image and self-esteem with adolescents and teens. You also know that I do not recommend these procedures lightly or without serious consideration for a child's total wellness—physical, psychological, and social.

Plastic surgeons have grappled with the ramifications of low self-esteem as a result of poor body image since the profession's inception. In 1932, Dr. Clarence Straatsma asserted that the goal of plastic surgery was to alleviate more than bodily pain. It was to relieve the mental anguish and potential inferiority complex that the realization of a defect could cause. Dr. Jacques Maliniak, the father of modern plastic surgery, wrote in his 1934 book *Sculpture in the Living*, "Once a child is aware of his disfigurement, he is at a disadvantage and predisposes to psychological disturbances. Correction helps restore the psychic balance."

Plastic surgery is not always the answer, and we'll address specific cases of when to say "no" and when to say "yes" in chapters 3 and 4. But it is one way to address physical concerns that are wreaking emotional havoc on kids. And for some physical deformities, it is the best solution: No amount of psychotherapy, no pill, and no consoling is going to put prominent ears in place or correct breast development in boys. "Dumbo" is no longer "Dumbo" when the ears are where they belong. "Girly Boy" disappears when male breasts are corrected.

Plastic surgery is not a panacea for teen angst. It is one arrow in the quiver of options, one spoke on the wheel of self-esteem. Sometimes just knowing that such an option is available is enough to make a troubled teen more secure with him or herself. Other times, it is part of a plan. And still other times, it is the entire plan.

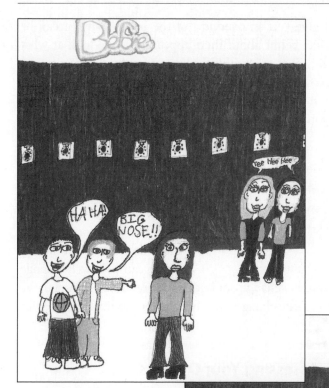

Before surgery the child is sad and isolated from her jeering peers.

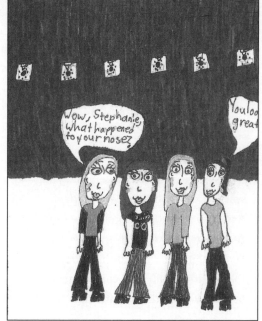

After rhinoplasty (nose surgery) her sense of self improves and she perceives a gain in peer acceptance.

23

In this chapter, I give you an overview of the basics of what can be done to help teens feel better about their appearance. We look at what can be done and why, what most ethical plastic surgeons won't do, and what should never be done. I also talk a bit about the differences between what was available ten to thirty years ago and what we can do today (e.g., your mother's nose job is not your teen's nose job, and a breast reduction done two decades ago is quite different from what's common now).

> We cannot exchange our bodies for brand-new ones, but we can make judicious and safe changes to certain parts and make peace with the rest.

I want to help you understand what can realistically be done for your teen and how quality-of-life surgery can positively change his or her life. We cannot exchange our bodies for brand-new ones, but we can make judicious and safe changes to certain parts and make peace with the rest.

Assessing Your Options

Let's assume that you've got the feeling that your teen may be suffering from body-image issues. You've observed the behavioral signs, and you've discussed them, perhaps using psychologist Dr. Glenn Pollack's techniques in chapter 1. You, of course, want to help your child. You've thought long and hard about it and may now be considering plastic surgery as a solution. So how do you go from listening and discussing body-image and self-esteem issues with your teen to offering a potential solution?

> The current generation of teens is only a mouse click away from everything they want to know about plastic surgery. And they see it on programs like *Nip/Tuck*, *Extreme Makeover*, and *I Want a Famous Face*. It is the clash between tabloid and reality that can add to a teen's own emotional suffering.

First, you should know that your child may already be aware of plastic surgery as a possibility. The current generation of teens is only a mouse click away from everything they

24

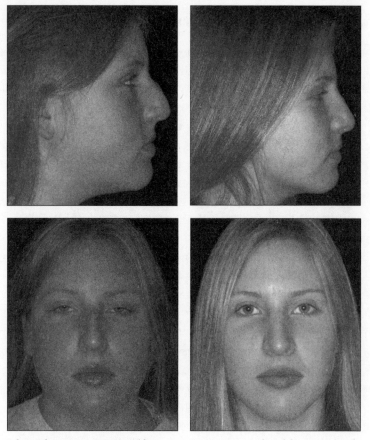

Rhinoplasty improving self-esteem. Patient seen after fifty pounds of weight loss. This is an example of combination therapies—surgery for structural change plus diet and exercise for overall well-being.

want to know about it. Some teens have gone as far as to get online consultations. Teens may have parents and grandparents who have had plastic surgery. They know friends or parents of friends who've had "work done." They see it on programs like *Nip/Tuck, Extreme Makeover,* and *I Want a Famous Face*—in fact, as I noted earlier, it is the clash between tabloid and reality that can add to a teen's own emotional suffering.

But teens are not able to get surgery without parental consent, and most do not have the financial resources to independently pay for it. So for surgery to be an option, the teen's parents need to come to the conclusion that it will be beneficial.

The Media's Take on Teenage Plastic Surgery

One of the biggest enemies of an adolescent's self-esteem is the media. It is also the matrix of some of the worst publicity about teenage plastic surgery. Often stories that masquerade as "information" are actually inflammation—blown-out tales of the minority of unethical doctors and all-too-willing patients.

The commercialization of cosmetic surgery in print media, on reality TV, on the Internet, and in advertising has produced an onslaught of messages that are easily misunderstood. Add to this mix the increasing number of non–plastic surgeons interloping into aesthetics, our societal obsession with beauty, and our desire for quick fixes, and we've created a perfect storm for the mushroom-like expansion of—and fascination with—plastic surgery in Gen X and beyond.

Plastic surgery is the Fertile Crescent for the media. After all, "if it bleeds, it leads." Media outlets often contact me because of my expertise. I become excited to speak on the real and substantive issues regarding teens and plastic surgery. But when I talk to the producers, I become dismayed. They want stories on teens desiring breast implants for graduation, or "mommy and me makeovers," or cosmetic disasters. I challenge them on the rationale behind presenting the most sensational stories as opposed to real stories of benefit. Their response: "It does not sell." They want the juicy stuff.

Once in a while, a story or article on the value of plastic surgery will appear. But unfortunately, the more lurid stories far outnumber the truly informative ones, and we in the plastic surgery community often have to defend the integrity of our practice. Many times when I've appeared on television to talk about the benefits of plastic surgery, the program has also invited someone as a counterpoint to argue against the necessity of the surgeries. This guest is usually a doctor who has little experience with teen patients but is a good PR person. We in the medical profession try to educate the media. But who wants to read about making people happy and average when we can feast on the catastrophic?

Sometimes a surgical solution is a fairly clear choice. For example, when a child has prominent ears and is suffering emotionally because of them, seeking an early surgical recommendation is the most prudent direction to take. Ears are fully developed by age 6, so any distressed teen or child older than 6 is a candidate.

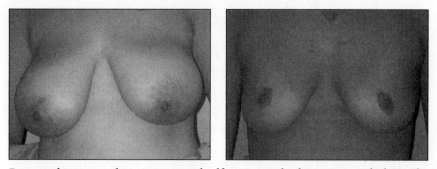

Breast reduction resulting in improved self-esteem and subsequent weight loss. The combination of therapies—surgery plus diet and exercise—improved her overall well-being.

Other situations may also readily point to a surgical solution, but the timing may not be right because the body is not fully developed. In these cases, the hope of surgical relief may be enough to buy psychological time for your teen until physically mature. For example, a nose problem should optimally be deferred until the face matures and balances itself, and breast asymmetry should be tackled once the breasts have stopped growing. Likewise, if boys have breasts, doctors should conduct a hormonal evaluation before surgery is considered. You do not want to perform surgery to correct a condition that may be occurring—and therefore recur—because of other factors (such as a hormonal imbalance or medication).

If you've discussed the option of plastic surgery with your teen and have concluded that a structural change will be beneficial, research the ideal surgeon for your child's issue. (For more on this important topic, see chapter 4.)

If the emotional toll on your child from the body-image issue has been severe, then psychiatric or psychological therapies might be needed in concert with the surgery. Plastic surgeons may presume to be amateur psychologists, and some psychologists may have their biases regarding the need for surgery, but in general, it can be quite beneficial for a teen and his or her family to work together with both types of professionals when the emotional scars from a physical problem run deep. Pediatric plastic surgeons value the insights and dialogues gained through psychology and psychiatry, and we recognize that by working as a team, we can evaluate and treat a teen both physically and emotionally.

There may also be situations in which surgery should be combined with a treatment other than psychotherapy, such as a diet and exercise program. Surgery might be the sole consideration for a teen with large breasts who is otherwise in ideal shape. But a girl with large breasts who is also overweight should consider addressing her weight issues prior to surgery.

The Motives behind Plastic Surgery

You may have read or heard stories of teenage plastic surgery in the media. If so, these were likely **not** the ones you need to know about to seriously consider surgery as an option for your child. You need facts, not sensationalism. The following are some real-life stories from my own patient files. They illustrate a wide range of issues and solutions.

- A 14-year-old boy had ears that stuck way out. His family thought his ears made him cute. His peers thought otherwise, and they let him know it. Names like "Dumbo" became part of his daily life. Once he left the safe haven of home each day and headed to school, the battle for survival began. The repeated taunts and jeers took over his life. His grades were suffering, and he was becoming reclusive. Should he have learned to live with what nature handed him? Would this added pressure have made him stronger or weaker? Should the family have considered a surgical correction at all? This teenager, when offered the opportunity for normalization of his ears through plastic surgery, jumped at the chance. Afterward, his grades improved, and he found himself becoming more and more socially confident. Today he is a normal, happy, and successful young man.

- A 16-year-old girl was a competitive swimmer. As she matured, her breasts became overly large. Two things happened as a result: swimming became more difficult, and she became known as the Dolly Parton of her eleventh-grade class. The physical limitations and social impositions were prompting her to withdraw socially. Was she too young to consider a breast reduction? Should she have struggled to compete in swimming or just given it up? Should she have tried to ignore the sexual innuendos? Her world was changing for the worse. Her parents sought out professional opinions about plastic surgery. The girl was evaluated by a psychiatrist to see if she could comprehend the risks, benefits, and outcomes of the surgery, and it was determined that she could. An endocrinologist also met with her to see that she was hormonally mature, and she was. She had the surgery and is back in the pool. She feels more "at home" in her body.

- A 15-year-old boy noticed that he was developing breasts, but he was too embarrassed to tell his parents. His behavior began to change. He refused to go to summer camp, he refused to go to the beach with his friends, he would not shower after gym class in school, and he was frequently in the principal's office for bad behavior. He also was taunted by his schoolmates for being "girly." Finally, it was brought to light that his sense of self was suffering because of a condition called gynecomastia (development of breasts in males). Should he have continued to avoid every situation in which he might have to take off his shirt and just hoped the condition would go away? The boy's pediatrician evaluated him for possible hormonal issues. When none were found, the doctor recommended a plastic surgical consult. The procedure to remove the abnormal breast tissue was straightforward and successful. The boy's physical and mental sense of self has healed, and now that vacation at the beach cannot come quickly enough.

- A 14-year-old girl had significant breast asymmetry. One breast was very small and underdeveloped, while the other was large and sagging. Her inability to wear a bra or bathing suit comfortably became increasingly problematic to the point of psychological depression, which was manifesting itself as irritable bowel syndrome. This complex problem required a procedure with two parts. One breast had to be uplifted and reduced while the other had to be made appropriately larger. Could this young girl accept the responsibility of a breast implant? Could she deal with the

Body Dysmorphic Disorder: When Normal Is Not Good Enough

The dread of every plastic surgeon is to miss the diagnosis of body dysmorphic disorder (BDD) and struggle in vain to take care of and please these never-to-be-satisfied individuals.

BDD is defined as a psychological disorder in which the affected person is excessively concerned with and preoccupied by an imagined or minor defect in appearance. At one time, anyone considering plastic surgery was thought to be neurotic and needed a psychiatrist. Until very recently, men who sought out cosmetic surgery were thought to have psychiatric problems. But actually, only about 1 percent of the population has BDD. It affects males and females equally. Those with true BDD do not believe themselves to be attractive on any level.

Symptoms of BDD often begin in adolescence after a child has internalized taunts and teasing and turned it into self-criticism. In some cases, BDD may be averted with proper interventions—both psychiatric and surgical—if caught early on.

Unfortunately, the true nature of the illness is sometimes not revealed until after the surgery, when all looks great but the patient still perceives an imperfection. The patient often requests further surgeries but is still never satisfied with the results. Consequently, the surgeon becomes more and more frustrated. The solution is no longer surgical.

As you read through the various chapters of this book, you will see references to BDD. I bring up the disorder in various contexts to give you a good understanding of how to decide whether or not your teen's desire for plastic surgery or dissatisfaction with his appearance is possibly a result of BDD.

scars of a breast reduction? She absolutely could, and she did. She is now very content with her body, and her IBS is gone. She is on the tennis team and is looking forward to college.

- A 13-year-old girl was singled out and picked on because her nose was significantly out of proportion to the rest of her face. She was called names and soon refused to go to school. Her parents tried to console her and promised her a "nose job" when she was 16. That hope for a different future was not enough, however. Her life was spinning out of control because of social ostracism. At last, her parents sought out a plastic surgeon for a consultation. It was clear that she was not fully grown and facially matured, but the emotional devastation of her current situation was overwhelming. Should her family have made her wait until she was 16, knowing she would continue to suffer emotionally in the meantime? Should she have been allowed the surgery at all? Knowing that she may need a second surgery when she was older, she and her family opted for a procedure that would refine her nose and balance it with her face. Her life improved. She became more secure and socially interactive. Her nose did change with age, but by the time she was old enough for a revision, she was so comfortable that she did not feel it was necessary.

- A 17-year-old high school senior had virtually no breast development. She felt masculine and was panicking about going to college. She was able to camouflage her chest in high school, but the dormitory experience frightened her. She worried so much that she stopped eating. Should she have just gotten over it and accepted what nature had given her? Would her eating disorder have eventually resolved itself? A plastic surgical consultation resulted in a pact between patient and surgeon: If she would do her part, he would do his. She entered psychotherapy to cope with her body-image issues and eating disorder, and a breast augmentation was planned for after high school with the agreement of her therapist. Although the timing might make it seem like it was a "graduation present," it was not that at all. It was a gift to normalize a feminine silhouette. It was planned in the transition period between one social experience (high school) and another (college). Having a comfortable body image allowed her to be successful—both academically and socially—in college. She is now a completely well-adjusted and happily married young woman looking forward to a lifetime of success and good self-esteem.

While these are examples from my practice, they're not isolated situations. Stories like these are happening all over the world, wherever teens are experiencing body-image issues. It is hard not to consider the benefits of plastic surgery when it can do so much for the right person at the right time.

The Role of the Plastic Surgeon

The ability to understand and appreciate teen body-image issues is what sets pediatric plastic surgeons apart from other plastic surgeons. A pediatric plastic surgeon shows a desire to interact with the teen and family and not dismiss him or her as overly sensitive or too young to be affected by the problem long term or just another case like all the others. The journey to a successful surgery begins with the cooperation of patient, parent, and surgeon. The feeling that we are all on the same team and a sense of trust is critical. This allows for fair discussions on when to say "yes" and when to say "no" or "later." It also opens the door to the possibility of other interventions like changes in nutrition, exercise, and dental care, and even psychotherapy.

Does your teen revere her body as a temple, or does she see it as a prison in which she's trapped? Does he take his looks in stride, or does he obsess? Have her views on her looks and related behavior overridden all other activities? If his behavior has changed recently, what was the catalyst? Is the teen justifiably concerned about a body part or consumed with vanity? What are the motivations for surgical correction? These are the questions that run through the mind of the plastic surgeon trying to sort out the ideal candidate versus the one who will never be happy with surgery and needs other interventions. We cannot immediately dismiss a child, but at the same time, we don't want to perform surgery on someone with a purely psychological issue such as body dysmorphic disorder (BDD).

As a pediatric plastic surgeon, I assume part of the responsibility of guardian of self-esteem. I need to be a part-time psychologist to navigate the waters of family indecision. I find myself advocating for a child when the parent is on the fence. It is my firm belief that a child who is derided for having big ears will never know peace until they are corrected. Parents may think their child looks cute with jug ears, but peers may view them—and vocalize their thoughts—differently. A teen with asymmetrical breasts will always be comparing herself to the norm and will never feel complete until she is balanced. I try to help parents understand the inner turmoil of their teenagers.

However, in being a child advocate, I don't always agree with the child. Many times I take the side of the concerned parents who feel their son or daughter is making a rash decision. By listening to children and respecting their feelings, I can oftentimes persuade them to wait until they have grown and developed more before making a decision. Agreeing to see a child again and revisit the option of surgery makes an adolescent feel that there is a light at the end of the tunnel and that someone is listening and cares.

As a problem solver, I will look at each patient as an individual and balance the physical with the emotional to reach a just decision. I also will discuss the risks, benefits, and outcomes. I have to be a voice of reason to many a teenager. Sometimes this is because of misconceptions a teenager has about what can be done. Teens may not understand, for example, that what a young celebrity did is not consistent with the standards of good medical practice. I do not perform breast implant surgery for purely cosmetic reasons before breast development is complete. I do not do breast reductions if the breasts are still growing. Almost all nose surgeries need to be deferred until the facial growth is complete. Procedures like liposuction are not substitutes for diet and exercise.

Also, there are some procedures that are not suited for teens at all. Among them is hair transplantation. Teenagers' balding patterns are not fully defined. I have seen many distressed teens with an early onset of hair loss. The reason the transplant procedure is not recommended for them is because the hair that is transplanted comes from regions of the scalp that retain hair. When the transplanted hair is placed into the balding areas, the job is done only temporarily, because as balding progresses—and it does until the person reaches his 30s or 40s (which is why I recommend waiting until then for the procedure)—the teen will be left with patches of hair and patches of baldness, as well as scars from where the hair was taken, especially if the overall pattern thins as well. The pharmaceutical industry is working hard on drug therapies to stop hair loss, and if it succeeds, it will be big news. At the present time, over-the-counter Rogaine and prescription Propecia are used with mixed results. As a surgeon, I do not want to place my patients on long-term drug therapies for cosmetic use. I refer them to dermatologists who work with these problems.

Decisions for teenage plastic surgery are family, and even extended-family, decisions. Many times I have met with the prospective patient and discussed options along with parents, siblings, and even grandparents. In my practice, I consider adolescents to be up to age 22, or until they graduate college. Most patients I see are still under parental control. The parents control the financial purse strings and therefore are part of the decision-making process.

When you care for a child, you are in it for the long haul. Adults seeking plastic surgery may come and go, but children continue to grow and mature, making follow-up visits very important. A pediatric plastic surgeon often becomes part of the extended family and serves as a resource for the patient throughout his growth and development. I once operated on a child with a cleft palate at age 1. At 13 she developed an unrelated problem, and her mother called me for advice. I arranged the neurosurgical consultation, and the procedure resolved a nearly devastating problem. Offering this kind of support is just part of being committed to kids and families. If your surgeon is not cut from that cloth, then he or she may not be the right one for you. Children need a significant amount of emotional support inside and outside the surgical arena. (See chapter 4 for tips on selecting a surgeon.)

Types of Surgeries

I am often asked what procedures I do most frequently. This is a complex question, because every patient presents his or her own issues. Each patient's problem requires a tailored resolution. This is partly why I view myself as a problem solver rather than simply a performer of procedures.

That being said, my most commonly performed surgeries on teens are:

- Otoplasty (ear surgery)
- Rhinoplasty (with or without chin and cheek augmentation)— facial balancing
- Breast reductions and breast-balancing procedures
- Excision of skin lesions and scar revisions

Other procedures that were previously performed primarily on adults have now entered the teen world. One of these procedures is the full-body lift needed to treat patients who have lost significant amounts of weight and whose skin did not shrink. Their "reward" for overcoming obesity is to be trapped in an unappealing envelope of loose skin. Breast lifts and body-lift procedures (tummy tucks, thigh lifts, etc.) are less common than those in the above list, but they are increasing as the obesity epidemic grows and teens take control of their health either on their own or with bariatric surgery.

There are other procedures that I perform less frequently but still consider on a case-by-case basis:

- Liposuction—usually on spot areas that have not responded after diet and exercise—for contouring (not as a weight-control treatment)
- Breast augmentation for reconstructive situations or in cases of severe psychological distress over lack of female development (not approved for teens under 18 except in these circumstances)

Procedures I do not do on anyone, young or old, include:

- Chest (pectoral) implants in boys
- Calf implants
- Buttock implants

Chest, calf, and buttock implants can cause irritation as the skin and muscles move and rub together, prompting the implants to shift, bulge, or even extrude through the skin. The implants also can result in infections. Unlike breast implants, which are either soft cushions of silicone or saltwater bags, the implants used in the butt, chest, and calves are solid silicone (Silastic). Because of their rigidity, they are prone to problems.

Implants of any kind, although safe and FDA approved, carry with them the burden of responsibility. They are foreign substances, although inert, and require due diligence, which means a lifetime of maintenance and possibly further surgeries to correct growth-induced changes or for replacement. Most implants reside comfortably in place and never cause problems.

The Most Common Plastic Surgeries

According to the 2009 report of the American Society of Plastic Surgeons' National Clearinghouse of Plastic Surgery Statistics, the most common surgical procedures performed in individuals younger than 20 were the following:

- Major procedures: rhinoplasty, male breast-reduction surgery, female breast-reduction surgery, and otoplasty—more than 100,000
- Minimally invasive procedures: laser hair removal, laser treatment for leg veins, skin treatments with chemical peels, and Botox—more than 200,000
- Breast augmentations—exceeding 9,000*

* This is for the 18- to 19-year-old group only.

They are usually the ones placed in static, or nonmoving, body parts—chin implants, for instance. Breast implants are the most "traditional" of implants and, for the most part, remain safe and comfortable (though they do require care over the years for safety reasons).

Implants are not the only way to increase the size of a body part. Fat grafting shows the promise of being a healthy and aesthetically pleasing alternative. There are new techniques for fat grafting that can be used to build up pectoral areas, calves, and buttocks, and, in the right situation, can provide benefit without the challenges of maintaining the implants. Research to evaluate these techniques as a possibility for breast augmentation is ongoing.

The Timing

When it comes to the timing of plastic surgeries, there are two things to consider: one, the timing in terms of development and, two, the timing in terms of recovery and transition.

Some types of plastic surgery should not be performed on a child until the affected body part has reached maturity. No doctor wants to operate on a still-growing body (unless it is under special circumstances like those I've discussed previously). Here is a look at a few areas of the body and when the timing is right to work on them:

- Ears (too prominent)—early teens and younger, usually beginning at age 6
- Face (disproportionate noses and chins) and male breasts—mid-teens
- Female breasts (too big, too small, uneven)—late teens
- Skin (moles and acne scarring)—any age

Because they're having surgery to deal with an area of their body that has caused significant distress, young people are generally reticent to announce it. For this reason, many choose to undergo surgery during long vacations or transitional social periods, such as between middle school and high school or high school and college. This timing consideration is important because it allows the child to enter the new social environment with a fresh start. First impressions are often lasting impressions, and deferring a surgery until a vacation period allows the teen to undergo changes and heal *before* reentering social situations. Another reason that having surgery during a long vacation can be ideal is because some sports and other school activities may need to be curtailed during the recovery. More on timing is addressed in the chapters on specific types of surgeries.

> Because they're having surgery to deal with an area of their body that has caused significant distress, young people are generally reticent to announce it. For this reason, many choose to undergo surgery during long vacations or transitional social periods, such as between high school and college. This allows the child to enter the new social environment with a fresh start.

Ongoing Communication

As you move forward with your decision for plastic surgery, it's important to keep in mind that communication doesn't stop at any point in the process, for it is just that—a process. The entire journey—deciding on the problem, working through the problem, and dealing with what follows—requires communication.

The Changing Landscape of Plastic Surgery

If you had plastic surgery years ago, you should know that much has changed. The surgery your son or daughter has will be very different than what you or your friends may have experienced years ago.

Reconstructive procedures like those for a cleft lip or palate, ear reconstruction, burn reconstruction, and trauma reconstruction existed in the '80s as they do today. Cosmetic surgeries were available, too, such as the nose job for the 16-year-old girl over the spring recess. Ear pinnings likewise have remained constant throughout my career.

But the way in which the surgeries are handled is different today than in the past. Instrumentation, lighting, anesthesia, and anatomic understanding have all evolved. The stage and its players are different too.

Most of the time, working through the process results in a successful outcome. However, sometimes the best intentions go awry. For instance, perhaps all the psychological and plastic surgical consultations have led to the decision for surgery, but then, the day of the surgery, the patient has a change of heart. I can recall two such circumstances that will forever reinforce that despite our best intentions as physicians and parents, we are all human and cannot account for every variable.

A preteen was all set for an otoplasty to pin back ears that were apparently bothersome. When the child was in the changing room, the game suddenly changed. He barricaded the door and refused to come out, saying he had changed his mind. Was this presurgery jitters or a true change of mind? We were at a crossroads. What to do? Talk him through it, force the surgery on him, or retreat for another time? Respect for the child was the priority, and the surgery was postponed.

Another young patient, a teen, was adamant about having her nose done—or so it seemed. She was fine in the admitting area and fine walking into the operating room and getting onto the operating table. Then the anxiety of her decision manifested itself in a crescendo of statements: "I do not think I want to do this" to "I do not want to do this" to "I really do not want to do this" to "Get me off this table now!" Obviously, the surgery was curtailed, and the teen was given time to sort out the right time and place for this particular solution.

Communication continues beyond the surgery as well. Some teens will need help dealing with the recovery and the adjustment to their new look. I had a teen patient who desperately wanted his ears pinned back. He was emotionally tortured at school. The surgery went very well, and afterward, he looked as normal and average as apple pie. Both he and his parents were delighted until he went back to school. He was unprepared for the comments that now centered on his surgery. He was deeply bothered by people speaking of his surgery. He needed further therapy to give him the psychological tools to deal with his new appearance and dismiss peer comments.

Judging a Surgery's Success

Any surgery that resolves the problem should be deemed successful. The surgeon's goal from the outset is for the procedure to be life-enhancing—for your teen to be happy with the outcome and to put the problem behind. When balance and harmony, both physically and mentally, are achieved, the patient and family find peace, and the surgeon feels he has performed his task well.

The Techniques

Techniques in the '80s were less sophisticated. Today, science is on our side. We have video-assisted equipment, like the tools used by orthopedic and laparoscopic surgeons. We can get into spaces and do certain surgeries with much smaller incisions—meaning the scars are much smaller as well.

Breast-reduction surgery, for example, can now be done with more discreet incisions. For most younger patients, the underneath scar (called the "anchor") has been replaced with the "lollipop vertical," a much more appealing scar for self-conscious youth.

Liposuction, too, has become much more refined. The advances allow it to be used successfully in some male breast reductions to even further reduce incisions and scarring and to allow for faster recovery. It can also be judiciously used for spot areas such as under the chin.

By using tissue expanders—basically deflated balloons placed strategically under the skin—we can stretch tissue (just as pregnancy slowly stretches the abdomen). We use this expanded skin to cover defects that are created when we remove burn scars and large, unsightly moles. In the past, a large skin graft would have been needed.

These technological advances go hand in hand with a greater understanding we now have of the anatomy and its response to surgery. The nose job today, for example, often uses an open approach, in which all the structures of the nose can be visualized; this allows for subtle refinements and repositioning rather than gross removals. Our understanding of facial balance has allowed for less radical nasal reduction procedures, meaning, for instance, a smaller nose refinement complemented with chin and/or augmentation.

Another area that has developed over the years is microsurgery, which has freed us to move tissue from one part of the body to another and allows for replanting of amputated parts and reconstruction of parts, like breasts after mastectomy. This is only the beginning. With breakthroughs in immunology, we will soon be able to transplant parts from other people. For reconstructive pediatric plastic surgery, this could mean ideal ear reconstructions when no ear is present, hand reconstructions, and even face transplants for those with burn injuries. In addition, tissue engineering may someday allow us to grow body parts from our own cells. Need a nose? Grow your own. Born without an ear? Grow one.

In the upcoming years, lasers will undoubtedly become more sophisticated and become bigger players in the surgical toolbox. Laser therapies have direct applications like cutting tissue without causing it to bleed, melting fat, and treating wrinkles; in the future, they also may have applications in becoming part of the solutions in treating obesity.

Computer Imaging

The greatest diagnostic development, for me, is computer imaging. It allows patients, families, and me to look at the problem together at the time of consultation. It is a real image in all views and not the familiar image seen in the mirror (which is actually the reverse of a photograph). My ability to morph structures on the computer image allows me to show the patient what I believe I can do. It also can clarify why some things should not be done. The computer surgery lets the patient see how he or she will look postsurgery. Many nose patients realize they need a chin augmentation when they see the balanced face put before them.

Bring On the Fat

The single biggest therapeutic breakthrough is our ability to use fat for augmentation. For years, clinical research has shown that fat can be used to enhance structures. It appears that fat assumes the character of the context tissue: if it is placed adjacent to bone, it feels like bone; into muscle, it feels like muscle; and into fat, it feels like fat.

I use fat grafting to augment chins and cheeks in teen patients. It allows me to avoid using implants in favor of the patients' own biological tissues. There is evidence that there are stem cells in fat that help to maintain the result. I have always avoided inserting chest implants in boys, as well as calf and buttock implants, because of the potential long-term consequences (discussed previously in this chapter). This technique of fat grafting may allow me to rethink this issue for those with real needs. There is also exciting work being done to research fat transfers for small to moderate breast augmentations. For some, this could eliminate the need for breast implants.

The Surgeons and the Patients

In addition to all of the procedural changes over the years, there is also another key difference in the world of plastic surgery today: The number of those who do the operations has significantly increased. When I became board certified as a plastic surgeon in 1982, there were a little more than 1,300 members. Now there are more than 6,000. Originally, only plastic surgeons practiced plastic surgery. Now there are Ear, Nose, and Throat (ENT) doctors who call themselves facial plastic surgeons as well as ophthalmologic surgeons and dermatologic surgeons adding the "plastic" moniker to their credentials. There is no regulation on who can use the name. It seems everyone now has a finger in the pie, vying for the moneyed procedures. Thus it has become increasingly important for you to research plastic surgeons carefully and choose a surgeon who is fully qualified to treat your teen's problem.

Today, more young people are having surgery compared to the 1980s, when plastic surgery was really just beginning to explode onto the scene. Back then, we were more timid about doing surgery on teens. Plastic surgeons who were new to the field were warned about operating on teen patients. Teens giving what today would be justifiable and acceptable reasons for surgery were dismissed as having BDD. Teen boys especially were red-flagged as psychologically problematic. Today, we understand that not all teens belong in this category, and we are better able to distinguish between the patients who will benefit from plastic surgery and those who won't.

3

When No Is the Answer

ALTHOUGH I HAVE SEEN the amazing life changes that can result from successful plastic surgical solutions for teens, I also know that there are times when "no" is the right answer. Or "not right now" or "let's wait and see." And certainly before a "yes" decision can be reached, there must be preparedness for a "no."

Parents are naturally protective of their children and often think with their hearts as opposed to their heads. It is almost instinctive for them to say "yes" more than "no." Similarly, children, especially teens, have a very hard time accepting "no" for an answer.

This chapter is devoted to helping you understand when "no" is the proper response. It also explores reasons that society and the media should demonstrate temperance and restraint, and it discusses what happens when the decision should have been against surgery but the teen "slipped through." Additionally, by eliminating the no's, this chapter sets the ground rules for who can be a "yes."

The Media's Message

"Plastic Surgeon Performs 35-Pound Liposuction on 12-Year-Old in His Office, Followed by 10-Pound Tummy Tuck. Says He 'Would Do It Again'!"

So flashes the headline in *People* magazine in fall of 2006.

The surgeon, the self-proclaimed "biggest fat-sucker in Texas," according to *People,* had his fifteen minutes of fame as he made the talk-show circuit with the young girl. His decision to do this risky surgery on such a young patient belied all the principles that most plastic surgeons live by. I, for one, feel that this preteen needed counseling and possibly weight-loss surgery before cosmetic surgery. Also, a procedure of this magnitude should never have been in an office setting. This tween was fortunate everything went well, as was the surgeon. The risks were huge; she could have had complications with anesthesia, bleeding, infection, and healing. This surgeon's decisions were far from mainstream practice. In this case, the answer should have been "no."

When teens are bombarded with tabloid blitzes about dramatic transformations, it is hard for them not to see plastic surgery as a real and easy option. They also can be influenced by peers who have had plastic surgery and might see it as a sort of rite of passage. Online consultations can further entice a teen to believe that plastic surgery is the correct path. These Internet sessions can present incomplete or misleading information that can be persuasive to teens as well as their parents. People tend to forget that plastic surgery is real surgery and therefore has real-life risks.

> When teens are bombarded with tabloid blitzes about dramatic transformations, it is hard for them not to see plastic surgery as a real and easy option. They also can be influenced by peers who have had plastic surgery and might see it as a sort of rite of passage.

Sorting Out the Issues

When parents are approached by their teen about plastic surgery, they need to ask:

- Why do you want the surgery?
- What are you trying to fix?
- Where did you get the impression that plastic surgery would help?

Asking these questions will help you begin a dialogue with your teen that is not immediately adversarial but shows that you are concerned about her and want to work as a team to resolve the issues that are causing her to look at plastic surgery as a potential solution. Your teen's answers will help you differentiate between a need and a want, though discerning which category his request fits into can be very difficult.

Parents, as a rule, try to do what is best for their children. They must fully evaluate something as significant as altering a body part and decide if it is in their teen's best interest. The idea of a surgery solving all you child's problems can be enticing, but the reality of his undergoing the knife can be daunting. You need to weigh the pros and cons.

The process is very much a buyer-beware scenario. You need to do your research and examine your child's situation carefully. If at anytime there is uneasiness with the concept of an operation, then the answer must be "no" or "not now" until issues behind the uneasiness have been resolved.

If you have a legitimate reason to defer or decline your teen's request for plastic surgery, then no amount of cajoling or pleading from your teenager should sway you. I encourage parents to be the first stopgap for teens seeking plastic surgery. If your initial thought is that there are other solutions for your teen's problem, then explore those solutions. If your teen really needs to lose twenty pounds, then focus on that as the key issue, and look for solutions less drastic than surgery. You don't want your teen to try to use plastic surgery as a cure-all.

You may decide that plastic surgery is not out of the question but that the timing is not right. Timing is a constellation of optimals. It may be that your child is not ready. Or it could be that her health is an issue—ideally we want optimal physical and emotional health before surgery. So sometimes the decision to forgo surgery is not a definitive "no" but simply a "not now." The beauty of quality-of-life surgery is its elective nature.

I encourage parents to sort out these possibilities before they seek a plastic surgeon's opinion.

Disagreeing with Your Teen

Disagreements between parents and teens over whether or not plastic surgery is the way to go are not uncommon. A teen may want the surgery, but his parents do not see the relevance, the need, or the benefit. Alternatively, parents may believe plastic surgery would improve their teen's life, but the teen is either ambivalent or against it. In situations like these, professional psychological help can be beneficial.

A teen may be well adjusted but legitimately bothered by an issue. A parental "no" without justification may be detrimental and cause significant family stress and dissention. Outside intervention could bring all sides together.

If a parent recognizes behavioral changes and believes plastic surgery may address the cause behind them, but the teen is nevertheless opposed, outside resources can help the teen see the benefit or, conversely, help the parent see that "no" is actually the best answer at this point in time.

Reasons to Back Away

Here are some important scenarios for choosing "no" or "not now":

- The teenager is not emotionally prepared.
- The teenager is not developed enough physically (for example, rhinoplasty should not be performed until the nose is fully developed, which generally happens between ages 13 and 16).
- There is a physical ailment that first needs to be addressed (see the next section).
- There is a psychological condition that must first be dealt with (see the next section).
- The parents are unable to pay for the surgery.
- The family finds the process of selecting a surgeon too complex, or they can't find one they're comfortable with (see chapter 4 for tips on choosing a doctor).
- The selected surgeon is not convinced that a procedure will be beneficial for the teen.
- Other treatments, such as a nutritional and exercise program, should be tried first.
- The teen is well adjusted and does not want surgery.

Physical Ailments and Psychological Conditions

If your child has general physical ailments, either acute or chronic, they need to be resolved or controlled prior to consideration of elective surgery. Weakened states of health can jeopardize healing and prolong recovery.

Conditions such as asthma, anemia (low blood count), and diabetes need to be treated to eliminate undue surgical and anesthesia risk. The patient should be free of illnesses like the flu prior to a procedure. Seasonal allergies also need to be under control before surgery can take place. Gastrointestinal problems such as Crohn's disease and ulcerative colitis must be thoroughly evaluated to determine the root cause and be under optimal control before surgery can be considered. Also, without question, cardiac conditions will preclude or delay any thoughts of surgery. In addition, certain medications used to treat irritable bowel syndrome—such as aspirin, which thins the blood and prevents clotting, and steroids, which impair wound healing—may in themselves be problematic for surgery.

If your child has psychological problems that are not a direct result of a physically correctable issue, then surgery must be rejected or at least deferred until such matters are resolved. Parents need to be aware that unless surgery will eliminate the root cause, your child's emotional turmoil will continue even after surgery. In fact, a surgery would likely only add to your child's burden because it would fail to meet his or her expectations.

In situations like this, a good plastic surgeon utilizes all his experience in dealing with a young person's emotional angst, and he can help you sort through the situation. If, for example, your child's problems are biochemical, then he or she will benefit more from seeing a psychiatrist for drug therapies and counseling than from seeing a surgeon. If you've noticed behavioral issues in your child, consider first that they may be triggered by nonphysical factors, like negative family dynamics. Your teen may say he or she desires aesthetic surgery because he or she may be unconsciously thinking that an operation will heal emotions that are in fact not related to a significant physical issue.

Anorexia and irritable bowel syndrome are disorders that have both physical and emotional causes. Resolution of these problems requires a team approach involving health disciplines outside of plastic surgery. However, when these disorders are the symptoms of a larger problem involving body image, plastic surgery should be part of the discussion because it could bring about improvement.

Another type of crossover ailment is body dysmorphic disorder (BDD), a condition characterized by an obsession about a physical flaw (real or imagined) that affects about 1 percent of the population. According to the *Diagnostic and Statistical Manual of Mental Disorders*, Fourth Edition (*DSM-IV*), "this preoccupation must cause significant distress or impairment in social, occupational or otherwise important areas of social functioning; and cannot be accounted for by another disorder such as anorexia nervosa" (American Psychiatric Association 2000).

As discussed in chapter 2, BDD symptoms often begin in adolescence. Because body image is so important in teens, BDD can lead to an unrealistic desire for aesthetic enhancement. Sometimes the physical issues bothering teens may in fact be real but are overblown in their minds, and this may or may not be true BDD. An experienced observer can tell the difference. If you suspect your child has BDD, it is important to refer him or her to a skilled

> Teens with undetected BDD could be traveling down the road toward plastic surgery addiction—they'll want to keep having surgeries because they'll never be satisfied. Good plastic surgeons do not want to operate on patients with BDD; they will avoid it at all costs.

psychiatrist who can help sort out the teen's worries and determine if surgery is justified or dangerous. Teens with undetected BDD could be traveling down the road toward plastic surgery addiction—they'll want to keep having surgeries because they'll never be satisfied. On the other hand, an incorrect diagnosis of BDD for a teen could mean he is deprived of a valuable procedure.

An experienced plastic surgeon often has good instincts about BDD, and believe me, good plastic surgeons do not want to operate on patients with BDD; they will avoid it at all costs. But sometimes even the best can be fooled and don't discover until after surgery that they are dealing with a patient with the disorder.

Most teens with body-image issues do not suffer from BDD; their negative emotions are simply out of proportion to the physical issue. When a teen's physical flaw is so internalized that it interferes with functioning, a psychiatrist should be consulted. The teen may not be suffering from true BDD, but the ramifications can be as significant, and a trained professional can help. People with BDD may also suffer from obsessive compulsive disorder (OCD), which causes such activities as excessive looking in mirrors and repetitive brushing of hair. But it's possible for a person to exhibit these OCD symptoms and not have BDD. According to Dr. Victor Fornari, chief of pediatric and adolescent psychiatry at Steven and Alexandra Cohen Children's Medical Center (formerly Schneider Children's Hospital) in Long Island, New York, anxiety disorders affect 10 percent of the population, OCD affects 3 percent, and true BDD, again, affects less than 1 percent.

Dr. Fornari and other psychiatrists say that BDD is overdiagnosed, and the media has bandied the term about so broadly that it is hard for parents to identify the problem. This means that when it comes to BDD, a do-it-yourself diagnosis does not work. Again, if you suspect that your child has an emotional or psychological issue that overrides any real bodily defect, seek the opinion of a credentialed psychiatric professional. This experienced doctor, along with a plastic surgeon, can determine if the psychological problem stems from a body issue that can be resolved through plastic surgery or if other measures are needed instead of or in addition to surgery.

The Physical–Emotional Grid

Psychologist Dr. Mark Gerstein and I have created an easy-to-understand chart that we call the physical–emotional grid to help you examine and understand your teen's body-image issues. Once you can classify his or her problems, you can begin to look for the solutions. Physical problems encompass issues that have an impact on bodily health. Emotional problems involve crises that affect mental health. The two types of problems are often intertwined—this is where the grid can be helpful.

"P" represents the physical and "E" the emotional.

P	P
E	E

If we were to draw an arrow from one letter in the first column to one letter in the second column, we could draw four possible arrows: from physical to physical, from physical to emotional, from emotional to physical, and from emotional to emotional.

P to P

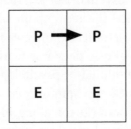

In a P-to-P situation, physical problems are causing more physical problems: large breasts are causing back pain and difficulty fitting into clothes or nasal problems result in breathing problems, snoring, and sleep apnea. There may also be emotional concerns related to the physical issues, but this scenario alone is reason enough to conclude that addressing the initial physical problem will solve the related issues. Thus, surgery is a viable option.

P to E

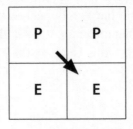

In this scenario, a physical flaw is causing an emotional crisis: ears that stick out result in torment at school, breasts on a boy bring social isolation, asymmetrical breasts on a girl cause severe embarrassment. Analysis here would conclude that correction of the physical problem will help the emotional issues, so surgery could be considered.

E to P

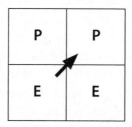

In this situation, emotional issues lead to physical troubles. Social isolation, for example, can cause a teen to view him or herself negatively, producing behaviors that can have physical effects. For example, if a teen sees herself as overweight, she may begin to starve herself. Although the teen is becoming physically ill, the root cause of the problem is an emotional one, not a physical one. Surgery here would only complicate her issues, making it a poor decision.

E to E

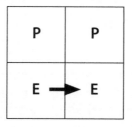

In this case, emotional issues, like depression, eating disorders, and even BDD, are at the core of the patient's problems. Teens with these emotional dilemmas may come to a plastic surgeon's office seeking surgery as a fix to perceived problems. They will claim to have a physical flaw or perhaps return to a surgeon asking for surgery "to correct another deformity." It is important to recognize that the underlying problem is psychological and seek the appropriate help—psychiatry or counseling.

Plastic surgery is most valuable in the P-to-P and P-to-E instances. It can be a useful adjunct in certain other situations, but only after the patient has had significant counseling.

Financial Constraints

Many parents are in agreement with their teen that he or she would benefit from surgery but must decline going forward because of the out-of-pocket expense. If this is the case, the parents and teen need to openly discuss the financial impossibilities of the surgery so that the teen can come to grips with the reality of a "no" answer. It's a hard "no" for the teen to accept, because the emotional or physical need for the surgery is still there. But an open conversation will let him know that it's not because his need isn't real but because the surgery cannot be managed financially. Teens need to accept the greater responsibilities of the family and perhaps understand that the surgery is not rejected but deferred.

Teens who are acceptable candidates for plastic surgery but have to put it off because of financial reasons can plan for their own future. At 18 years of age, they can legally proceed with surgery without parental consent. They can plan by working and saving and even asking for help from family members. Certain teens at 18 may also be able to take on the responsibility of borrowing independently.

See chapter 5 for information on weighing the costs.

Operating on Teens

The American Society of Plastic Surgeons (ASPS) has no official position on plastic surgery for teenagers. As with any surgery, parental consent is required for any teen under 18. The society "advises parents to evaluate the teenager's physical and emotional maturity and believes that individual cases merit careful evaluation under the guidance of a plastic surgeon certified by the American Board of Plastic Surgery." A briefing paper that is available on the organization's Web site (see the resource guide at the back of the book) outlines guidelines for teenage plastic surgery. The ASPS suggests that surgery is most beneficial when the teen has initiated the request, has realistic goals, and is sufficiently mature for surgery.

Reasons Why a Surgeon May Say No

Many plastic surgeons are wary about operating on the adolescent population. This is why there are subspecialists who have gained insight into this patient group. That said, responsible surgeons are looking for red flags as well as green lights.

Parents may consult a plastic surgeon's office only to find that their teen is denied the surgery. The following are reasons—many of them based on subjective impressions—surgeons turn away some teens.

- **The teen has other medical conditions.** Plastic surgery is real surgery with risks and a recovery period. It is, for the most part, elective, so timing can be planned and adjusted. Patients must be in optimal physical and mental health. If there are outstanding or untreated medical problems, the procedure cannot be done. All patients should have medical clearance from their pediatricians that is honest and truthful—no matter how great their desire to have the procedure.

  I once operated on a teen who came to me because another surgeon had performed a nose job on her with a poor result. I corrected her problem and felt very satisfied with the outcome. She had reservations and wanted more to be done. A red flag went up. A closer look at her medical history revealed that she was not honest about her surgeries and that she had received multiple operations on her nose in the past, each from a different surgeon and each creating more problems.

  I did not agree to operate further. Instead, I suggested she seek psychiatric help. She thanked me and left the office. She did not seek the help I recommended. She would periodically request appointments in the office but was told that without psychiatric counseling she would not be seen. Plastic surgeons rely on truthfulness and can be misled by patients with an overriding need to have a procedure done. Certainly this young girl needed psychiatric help, which is what I encouraged her to find. Because of situations like these, we strive to rule out potential patients who have other medical problems.

- **The teen is unwilling to change habits.** Each surgeon has criteria regarding habits that she is comfortable with. I personally do not operate on smokers, because smoking compromises healing. Other habits like excess alcohol and drug use will set up risks and should be red flags. Teens who want the surgery must be willing to alter their habits.

- **The parents are emotionally manipulative.** The plastic surgeon may sense that the parents are the principal drivers in the decision process for their teen's plastic surgery. Maybe a nose job is a rite of passage—all family members have had it, and they do not want their child to be different. Perhaps they are embarrassed by their child's prominent ears or are trying to be proactive. If the decision is not truly the teen's, then the surgery runs the risk of having physical success but emotional failure—which is why the surgeon would turn it down.

  One time I operated on a high school sophomore with ear asymmetry; both ears stuck out, and one did so much more than the other. This teenager was anxious to have them corrected. The procedure went well and he was happy, but his mother was less so. In her mind, the ears were not identical. This was true. It was explained to the patient, mother, and father at the initial consultation that the ears were different to start with and, though they would be much improved after surgery, they would not be a matched set. He was ready to move on with his life, but his mother was pushing for another procedure to further attempt to match the ears—even before the swelling was gone from the first procedure. I felt that we needed to allow time for the ears to heal, and I was confident that the teen would continue to be satisfied. The patient agreed, but the parents were still unhappy. However, I would not operate on this child until he had healed and decided he wanted the surgery himself. The parents may have pursued further operations with another surgeon; I don't know.

- **There is dissent within the family.** Pediatric plastic surgery is often a group decision. If a teen is under age 18, parental permission is required. It is possible that the teen wants the surgery and the parents do not or vice versa. Or the parents may disagree with each other. A surgeon sensing dissention will reject or defer the patient.

- **The teen or family has unrealistic expectations or is unable to comprehend the procedure, risks, and outcomes.** In the course of the consultation, it may become apparent that the desires are greater than what can be achieved. Patients and families who bring in celebrity photos or mocked-up photos from other offices can trigger red flags. Regardless of any detailed discussions we may have had, if I feel that what I can realistically do is not what the patient or his family desires, then I will politely say "no."

Sometimes what the patient or family wants runs counter to good surgical aesthetic judgment. In these cases, the surgeon will decline to operate. Likewise, when a surgeon reviews the risks with a patient, and the patient seems uninterested in understanding or accepting those risks, the surgeon will likely make the right decision and back away from what is potentially a problem patient. The patient and his family must be aware of limitations and the potential for complications or delays in healing. Things do not always go as planned. There must be trust between surgeon and patient and family in order to resolve any problems.

I recently saw a 19-year-old girl with breast asymmetry. One breast was very large, and the other was measurably smaller; both were sagging more than a teen's breasts should. Structurally, I felt she was an excellent surgical candidate. As I started to present options to her, which included uplifting the smaller breast and reducing the larger breast, she blurted out, "I want implants!" She was a tall girl and an athlete, and I was not averse to considering implants to balance her breasts to the rest of her body. However, the more the discussion progressed, the more fixated she seemed to be on very large implants. She was more concerned with the size of the implants than she was willing to listen to my expertise on what would look harmonious. Additionally, she wanted the surgery two weeks prior to going back to college in another state. This presented multiple red flags. She did not comprehend the procedure and would not listen to options. She was not allowing time for recovery. I did not conduct the procedure; my recommendation was to defer to a time when she could and would comprehend the surgery and recover fully.

■ **The teen is unable to accept recovery or commit to recovery limitations.** When a prospective patient doesn't want to allow time for recovery, it is a big red flag. Teens do not want their lives disrupted. It is part of the quick-fix, "I want it now and on my terms" mentality. It is difficult for some teens to grasp that "cosmetic surgery" is still real surgery. Patients often feel good soon after the surgery and will not listen to the cautions given to them about healing. If, in the course of a consultation, the teen is reticent about accepting the recovery period, then the procedure should be delayed or deferred. Similarly, if the potential patient's schedule won't allow for a full recovery period, this can be a red flag to the surgeon that this procedure is not a priority at this time in the teen's life and should be deferred.

Once, I evaluated and planned to operate on a teen who had lost a significant amount of weight and desired the excess skin to be removed from his abdomen. He was a good candidate for the procedure. He was anxious to have the surgery over the summer prior to entering college, which was logical. All seemed to be going as planned until I discussed the time for recovery. He could not accept the restrictions; in fact, he turned belligerent. He stated that he was "a kid and needed to have fun." This became a war of words. Because compliance seemed to be an issue, I sent him away, telling him to return only when he was mature enough to grasp the gravity of the surgical solution he wanted.

■ **The surgeon feels defensive.** There are times when parents or teens will bring in reams of Internet material and challenge every statement the surgeon makes during their visit. This approach places the physician on the defensive and interferes with a healthy dialogue. I am not talking about patients who do their research and come in with questions. I am talking about patients who are looking for negatives. This kind of doctor–patient relationship is not healthy and should be terminated before problems ensue. Sometimes the chemistry between the parties is not right, and, without blame or prejudice, the relationship should be discontinued.

There is an expression that "good judgment comes from experience, and experience comes from bad judgment." As a plastic surgeon, I often make the judgment to say "no" to a teen and his family. The reasons usually fall into the categories I have defined above.

The plastic surgeon is, by experience, an amateur psychologist. If he is ethical and professional, he is actively looking for the red flags. Everyone wants a successful outcome, and no one wants problems, especially long-term ones. We want our patients to be the best they can be for themselves, not for others or to look like others, or to feed a need that stems from undiagnosed psychological issues.

A good surgeon will say "no" as often as he says "yes." Saying "no" used to be easier when the surgery was riskier and had variable results. Progress has become a double-edged sword. Surgery is now safer and the results are predictable. This means that it is more important than ever to take your teen's health in hand and listen to a professional if he suggests waiting or forgetting about it altogether.

When 'No' Is Really 'Not Now'

There are circumstances when "no" is the answer at a given point in time but not necessarily definitive. Here are some examples:

- If the need is there and the only obstacle is scheduling, then deferring to a mutually agreeable time can turn a "no" into a "yes."
- Parents may see the benefits of the procedure but need time to financially prepare. A discussion with the teen will often buy the time needed.
- If there are medical issues (physical and/or emotional) that need to be resolved first, then a team approach by multiple medical professionals may allow for a happy ending via surgery at a later, safer time.
- Open discussions with families can sometimes resolve disputes and dissentions and pave the way for reconsideration at a later time.

Reasons Society Should Say No

A perfect storm is brewing. Our youth-oriented society has put teens in the more-faster mode, and many are not afraid to seek plastic surgery with this approach. The era of managed care in medicine has driven many physicians into the world of cosmetic surgery—but without proper training. Compound this problem with the heavy advertising for plastic surgery and add in the tabloid media stories, and the witches' brew equals disaster.

The American Society of Plastic Surgeons tries hard to regulate and educate its members to maintain the highest standards. It censures and disciplines members who violate the ethical bylaws. However, the society only has jurisdiction over its own roster. It cannot control the interlopers. Anyone with a medical license can in theory practice plastic surgery and claim to be a plastic surgeon. As long as society, and especially the media, allows and promotes the drama of plastic surgery, and there is no discrimination between who is an expert and who is not, the burden is heavy on the prospective patient and family to find a true expert. Until we as a society recognize the experienced surgeons, the patient is vulnerable. Until there is a regulation of the reality programming and the tabloid media that glorifies the celebrities there will be limited positive influence on a teen's thinking and emotions about plastic surgery.

We should be interested in the benefits that reconstructive surgery offers and respect the decisions of those experts who follow the moral high ground.

We as parents and physicians should say "no" when our teen's desire for change is frivolous—when his or her reasons are not sincere or he or she is doing it for someone else. We should carefully evaluate who is a good candidate and who is not. Once the red flags are up and the poor candidates separated out, then it becomes apparent who will benefit from plastic surgery.

I have spent my life in pursuit of excellence. I am not like and will never equate myself with the doctors on programs like *Dr. 90210* and *I Want a Famous Face*. I believe they exploit the audience and trivialize what we do. We as physicians stand on the shoulders of those who have practiced before us. We owe it to them and those who will come after us to do the right thing.

I try to educate the public about the true value of plastic surgery as quality-of-life surgery. My professors used to remind us that "we are playing cards with patients' chips." They held us to the concept that we had a responsibility to physicans past and physicians of the future. I may be on a bit of a soapbox here, but I want to stress this aspect of teenage plastic surgery, and if I overemphasize it, so be it.

> Plastic surgery is not for everyone, and it should not be reduced to a media circus.

Plastic surgery for teens is a real quality-of-life solution. Again—and this cannot be overemphasized—plastic surgery is not for everyone, and it should not be reduced to a media circus.

Final Thoughts

Use the red flags described in this chapter to evaluate your teen's situation yourself, and if necessary, take care of your teen in the long term by denying his or her heart's desire in the short term. Say "no" when it is appropriate, and you may be saving more than money—you will be ensuring your teen's emotional and physical well-being.

4

Moving Forward with Surgery

ONCE THE LINES of communication are open and you and your teen have determined together that a plastic surgical solution to a specific problem is the path to pursue, your attention must now shift to ensuring that your teen has a successful outcome. You did not come this far in the decision-making process to cut corners here. You've been cautious in deciding to go forward, so now you must be just as careful in making the right decisions for your teen to have a successful and healthy outcome.

Your next step is to choose your surgeon and where the surgery will be done. It is important during the entire process to continue to maintain open dialogues with your teen. The final decision should be based on objective criteria and the subjective impressions of both you and your teen. At every step of the way, consider your teen's feelings and intuitions. Keep talking. No one was ever harmed by too much communication!

Both you and your teen need to feel safe and secure in this choice. You may each get different impressions that need to be sorted out. Even the way you make the initial selection for a consultation needs to be discussed. Who chooses the surgeon? Is he or she a referral from a friend at school who had a similar surgery performed? Is he a family friend? Is he a surgeon who worked on an acquaintance on an unrelated body part? Did he appear in a magazine you saw? Although you as the parent may be doing most of the legwork, your teen needs to be present through the entire process. Otherwise, he or she may feel that decisions are being made behind his or her back.

You should expect good communication and support from your surgeon. Your plastic surgeon should be on your side regarding the impact the problem is having on your child's life and in finding the best possible solution to your child's problem. If he is not, find another surgeon.

Your plastic surgeon is the "captain of the ship." He is in charge of your teen's care throughout the process of his particular surgical solution. So choosing the right plastic surgeon is critical.

You want the best doctor for the job, and if that means traveling, then do so. But remember that if your surgeon is far away, follow-up is more difficult, and if there are any complications, the distance can be a problem. Look for excellence in your area before searching afar. I do not believe that plastic surgery tourism (traveling abroad for cheaper deals) is appropriate for teen plastic surgery. Too many variables are completely out of your control. I am not trying to scare you by saying that your plastic surgeon has your child's life in his hands; this is just the reality of *any* surgery.

> Kids want to act quickly; they are often impulsive by nature and have an air of immortality that puts them in denial that anything can go wrong. This is where the responsibility of the parent is crucial. Parents need to be active in the process of choosing who and where.

The decision about a surgeon is best made after you've gathered all the facts and then digested the information. Kids want to act quickly; they are often impulsive by nature and have an air of immortality that puts them in denial that anything can go wrong. This is where the responsibility of the parent is crucial. Parents need to be active in the process of choosing who and where. They will sense which surgeon and office staff truly care about their child—which office shows empathy for their situation and will go to bat for them (including checking on insurance coverage), which office makes sure the preoperative information is correct and that the family understands the procedure, and which office will call after surgery to check on the patient and offer help and advice (this is a major plus).

You should not make a spontaneous decision about a surgeon. Remember: "Act in haste, repent at leisure." The following are important criteria you must first consider. Take these lists with you for easy reference. Do not be embarrassed to refer to them during a consultation. As the saying goes, "An educated consumer makes the best customer."

Do's and Don'ts in Selecting a Surgeon

1. **Check the credentials.** There are many specialties that dabble in plastic surgery and many doctors who will call themselves plastic surgeons. *Only doctors who have been certified by the American Board of Plastic Surgery are truly plastic surgeons.* You can access the American Society of Plastic Surgeons Web site at www.plasticsurgery.org; there you will see that all ASPS members are board certified plastic surgeons. You can also see if your surgeon has a special interest in adolescents by asking if he belongs to the American Association of Pediatric Plastic Surgeons.

   There are many new societies and boards that are smoke screens, created to lend credibility to those who are not certified by the American Board of Plastic Surgery (ABPS). Only ABPS is recognized by the American Board of Medical Specialties. You should be cautious if, when researching a specific surgeon, all you find is something saying he has certificates from "cosmetic surgery boards and societies." Be aware also that there are physicians who are certified in other disciplines who will state that they are "board certified" without specifying what they're board certified to practice. Board-certified plastic surgeons are proud of their accomplishment and openly display their credentials. They will gladly discuss their training and certification with you.

   Similarly, don't be fooled by false advertising and misleading Web sites. The Internet is poorly regulated and filled with misinformation and half-truths. If you surf different Web sites looking at "before" and "after" pictures, be aware that the photos shown are probably the best results and may not even belong to the physician who's claiming them.

2. **Meet the surgeon.** There is no substitute for a face-to-face consultation. When you go to visit a surgeon, bring your teen along with you, and retain a sense of calm. Advise your teen that you are fact-finding and gathering information. Many times the teen can be swept away at first blush and ready to book without a lot of thought. Your teen may need your parental due diligence to help look before leaping.

Also, as stated before, plastic surgery is a visual specialty and therefore pre- and postoperative photography is the custom. So prepare your teen for the likelihood that he or she will have pictures taken; this heads-up is especially important if he or she is shy or easily embarrassed by the area in question. Some surgeons send their patients to independent studios for pictures. I personally abhor this. In this world of digital photography and archiving, I feel that photography of such a sensitive nature should remain in the privacy of the office. Note that depending on the type of procedure, photography and imaging may be done as part of the initial consultation. For breast reductions and certain nasal surgeries the photographs are often sent to the insurance companies for documentation.

I once saw a patient who had initially gone for a nasal surgery consultation elsewhere. He was sent to a studio for photos, delaying any visual impressions until a later date. He had functional as well as aesthetic concerns. The plastic surgeon never even offered to inquire about insurance coverage for the functional aspect. I was able to use my computer imaging system to show him my aesthetic plan, and with the appropriate documentation, he was able to get partial insurance reimbursement for the breathing aspect. His parents pursued the most beneficial path for the teen and did their due diligence in selecting a surgeon, resulting in a successful surgery and insurance coverage they would not otherwise have had.

The following are some tips for your consultation:

- **Ask in advance if there is a charge for your consultation.** Sometimes there is a charge, although, like me, many surgeons do not charge for consultations. Patients are consumers and are trying to evaluate and formulate. I do not want to lose the opportunity to meet new patients because they have run low on funds for consultations. There are surgeons who will charge a consultation fee but deduct it from the surgical fee if the patient books, and there are others who feel that their time is valuable enough to charge a fee for that alone. This is a very personal decision and bears little on the quality of the work.

- **Do not be confrontational—after all, the surgeon is sizing you up as well.** You do not want to appear to be a difficult or uncooperative client. If the surgeon feels disinclined to work with you, he is not obligated to do so. Likewise, if you find the surgeon not to your liking, you are under no obligation to proceed. Having a solid rapport is key to the entire process, especially if there are some bumps in the road later.

- **Upon meeting a surgeon, politely ask about his experience with adolescents.** There are subspecialists, like me, who are experts in working with this group of patients and make it a major component of their calendar. On the other hand, there are those who feel that a nose is a nose and a breast is a breast and look at your child as just another case. This approach could work if there are no problems, but what happens when your child needs a little emotional TLC? Are the surgeon and office prepared to give it?

- **Ask about the surgeon's experience with the procedure you are interested in.** There are surgeons who have specific areas of expertise (noses, breasts, ears, body contouring, etc.), and it's in your best interest to find a doctor who has done many times over the procedure you are seeking.

- **Ask if you may have a second visit if more questions arise.** It is important that you not feel rushed and all your questions are answered.

- **Let your teen ask questions, and observe the interaction.** Is this surgeon "kid friendly"? Is your teen comfortable in this office environment and with the surgeon? In the course of the consultation, note whether the surgeon is speaking to you or your child. Teens can feel left out of the process if the surgeon seems to bypass them in conversation. Also keep in mind that the consultation can be intimidating for your teen. He or she is probably embarrassed about openly discussing the problem, especially if it pertains to a sensitive area like breasts or if it has been a source of ridicule. How the surgeon handles this sensitivity is a clue to what you can expect from the surgeon throughout the process.

- **Ask to see before-and-after photos.** Plastic surgery is a visual specialty. Make sure your surgeon can provide many examples, and ask to see average results, not just the showcase ones!

- **Ask if there are patients you can speak with.** If your surgeon hesitates, be concerned.

- **Meet the staff.** You will be interacting with them more than you think, so you should know them—and they should know you. Be observant. Is the office clean? Is your child the only child in the waiting room? Are the administrators and nurses enthusiastic about the presence of children in the office, or are they just tolerant?

- **Ask where the surgery is performed and who is involved (assistants? nurses? anesthesiologists?).** I discuss this in greater detail in the next section.

- **Ask the critical question about cost.** Do not be ashamed to bring it up; it is an important component of the initial consultation. What are the office policies regarding payment and the possibility of insurance reimbursement?

3. **Find out where the surgery will take place.** Part of the comfort level for your teen will involve the facility where the surgery will be performed. Plastic surgery has become very sophisticated; anesthesia has as well. The net effect is that most procedures are

done on an ambulatory basis. This means that there are various venues where surgery can be performed. Some surgeries are performed in an ambulatory pavilion of a hospital, others are done in a freestanding ambulatory facility, and still others are conducted in a surgeon's office. Consider the following points about the facility and the people working with your surgeon:

- **All facilities must conform to certain safety standards.** Hospitals and ambulatory surgical centers are certified by the Joint Commission (formerly known as the Joint Commission on Accreditation of Healthcare Organizations, or JCAHO). Office operatories should be certified by the American Association for Accreditation of Ambulatory Surgical Facilities (AAAASF). This is mandatory in some states and voluntary in others. You will need to check to make sure you see the certificate of accreditation. This ensures that the appropriate safety precautions are met. (See the resource guide at the back of this book for help on finding certified facilities.)
- **You need to enquire about the anesthesia.** Will there be a board-certified anesthesiologist? This is important because some surgeons use certified registered nurse anesthetists (CRNAs). This means that an additional burden of responsibility is placed on the surgeon, as he becomes the only physician and assumes a greater overall role in the total care. Because young patients are often undergoing anesthesia for the first time, I prefer to use pediatric anesthesiologists who are board certified and trained in this subspecialty.
- **Know the backup plan if your child is delayed in going home.** Will the facility and staff accommodate your child if he is not ready for discharge by the end of the day? Some facilities are not equipped for overnight stays or late stays. You need to know what happens if this is the case. Is your child transferred to a hospital? Some offices arrange for overnight nursing care in a hotel; are you comfortable with this?

Picking the Right Plastic Surgeon: Red Flags and Green Lights

Red Flags

- The office is not accommodating to your teen's schedule. Most offices that deal with children are sensitive to school schedules.
- The office is devoid of evidence of involvement with children and adolescents. There should be some other children in the office.
- The staff is ill at ease with an entourage. Teens will obviously come with their families, and the best offices are usually prepared.
- The surgeon does not speak directly to your child. Physicians who specialize in children like to interact with them.
- The surgeon is reluctant to show before-and-after photos or provide patient references. Surgeons love to show off their work; if this surgeon is not, beware!
- The staff is not receptive to questions. The patient is your child. You must be totally comfortable with the environment.
- The surgeon puts pressure on you to book the procedure. You have a right to take your time until you're certain.
- The surgeon minimizes the recovery. Plastic surgery is still real surgery and, like any surgery, requires healing time.
- The surgeon is offended by second opinions. A secure plastic surgeon welcomes second opinions, as they reinforce his own treatment plans.

Green Lights

- From the initial phone call, the office is inviting.
- The staff is very comfortable with the presence of children and their families.
- The surgeon interacts well with your child.
- The surgeon is happy to show you examples of his work.
- The surgeon is pleased to have you return for a second visit to answer any further questions.
- There are other children in the waiting room.
- The office is accommodating to children's schedules.
- The surgeon is very comfortable with all questions from you and your child.
- The surgeon does not pressure you to schedule surgery.
- The surgeon and office are honest in explaining the time needed to recover.
- The surgeon welcomes your seeking a second opinion.
- The surgeon is truly interested in making a difference in your teen's life.

Next Steps

You and your teen have met the surgeon and formulated an impression. Now it's time to reflect and discuss. Are your impressions the same? Are they positive or negative? If you are both on the same page, the next step is easier. If your impressions are positive, you can make a plan to go forward. If your impressions are negative or you disagree, then more family discussion is critical, as further investigation and consultations are most likely necessary.

The following checklist can help you decide if you're ready to move forward with the surgeon you're considering. Can you answer "yes" to all the below criteria?

- Did this surgeon listen to my child and explain things to him or her as well as me?
- Do I believe this surgeon will guide us through the recovery and be there for us if there is a problem?
- Are his goals specific so that our expectations do not exceed reality?
- Is our decision thought out, or have we made it in haste due to our desire to fit it into his busy schedule?
- Are we comfortable with the staff and the facility chosen for the procedure?

Now comes the leap of faith. All your research has led you to the decision to go forward with the procedure and with the chosen surgeon. This is a good time to reflect on the entire process and ask yourself the following questions:

- Have we, as a family, recognized a specific problem, and are we convinced that surgical correction will be helpful?
- Is the decision based on my teen's desire for change, and is my teen still well motivated?
- Do we have a realistic expectation of the results?
- Are we prepared for the recovery process? Have we planned for the required time and resource commitments? Will someone be home with my child during recovery? Does my child show a willingness to adjust his or her lifestyle during recovery?

- Am I comfortable with the surgeon when he outlines the procedure? Do I believe what he says is logical, even if it is different from what I was thinking before the consultation?

Final Thoughts

Your choice of surgeon is critical. Try to avoid using professional referral services that you may see advertised. Most services are subscribed to and paid for by surgeons, which means the services aren't unbiased. Avoid being seduced by advertisements, advertorials, and other public relations products in general. A good surgeon will have a reputation to stand on. Make sure your surgeon is who he says he is—legitimately board certified and trained in the area you need. Also, don't let a surgeon rush you into a decision. You want to make sure that "all your ducks are in a row." Most teen plastic surgeries are elective and can be scheduled at times that are comfortable for all involved.

Evaluate your experience at each level, from the initial consultation to the pre-op evaluation. Getting to "yes" is a big step, but it is only the first step in the process to bring a successful resolution to the problem that brought you here.

Review this important chapter thoroughly. Digest the criteria here, and bring copies of the checklists to your appointments. Your child's physical and emotional welfare depend on your choice of surgeon. The successful outcome of your teen's plastic surgery relies on many things, but the most important component is a board-certified, responsive, caring, and skilled surgeon.

I can't emphasize enough that you should take your time deciding and use all the information you can collect to help your decision. When I see a family who has taken the time to do their "homework," I see a team who is willing to work toward the best possible surgical result for the teen.

Review the Consultation Cheat Sheet box for an easy reference on what to look for during your first appointment with a surgeon. Again, don't be afraid to copy these pages and bring them (or the book) to your consultation. If a surgeon is unhappy or threatened by them, that is a definite red flag.

Consultation Cheat Sheet

Ask the following questions when you meet a surgeon:

- Are you certified by the American Board of Plastic Surgery?

- Are you a member of any pediatric societies like the American Academy of Pediatrics or the American Association of Pediatric Plastic Surgeons?

- What percentage of your patients are children?

- What procedures do you perform most frequently?

- Are you involved in continuing medical education to stay current?

- Do you have resources to seek out if you need help with any problems you may encounter?

- Where do you perform the surgery?

- Is the facility certified? Is it equipped to handle children? What happens if my child cannot go home?

- Who do you work with? Who assists you with the surgery? Do you do it all?

- Who performs the anesthesia?

- How long is the surgery?

- What is involved in the recovery process?

- Are there charges for follow-up visits?

- Are you available for questions after the surgery?

- Will you be around during the recovery, or do you have a vacation planned during that time?

- Can we see examples of your work?

- May we speak to patients of yours who have had our procedure?

5

Weighing the Cost

YOU'VE MADE THE DECISION that surgery on your teen would be beneficial to his or her overall well-being. After weighing all the physical and psychological ramifications and researching and selecting the best surgeon, you want to move forward.

The next question I always hear is, "Will my insurance cover the surgery?" This is where the wheels frequently come off the wagon. We, as physicians, see the emotional impact that body-image issues can have on teens. We recognize that this emotional angst can create other physical and psychological problems. We are patient advocates and agree that our patients often "need" the procedures. Your child is suffering, so you expect at least partial, if not complete, coverage from your insurance provider.

But the insurance world does not generally see plastic surgery the way we do, and getting insurance companies to cover it is difficult, when not impossible. Insurance companies recognize that emotional issues are significant, but unfortunately, they would rather pay for psychiatric care and drugs than pay for the surgery that could eliminate the root cause of the problem. This chapter gives you insight on what to realistically expect from your insurance provider and some suggestions for obtaining the necessary funds.

Cosmetic Surgery Tourism

Don't fall prey to the lure of cosmetic surgery tourism. The "destinations" in this budding industry are offshore surgery centers that offer cheap procedures combined with vacation packages.

The dangers of this practice are twofold.

First, once you leave American soil, you lose your legal rights. In other words, American medical malpractice laws do not apply.

Secondly, complications resulting from offshore surgeries can become difficult and expensive to fix. If your teenager has work done at one of these offshore locales and develops a problem related to it, it will be difficult to find an American surgeon who will pick up the responsibility for it. If your child has postsurgical problems while still away from the United States, you'll be paying for food, lodging, and other expenses while the problems are being resolved.

Cost versus Value

As you consider the cost of plastic surgery, first and foremost remember that cheaper is not better. Quality comes at a price.

For your child you want the best. The decisions you make can have lifelong ramifications. A successful outcome means that your child can put the original issue behind him and that his life goes on better than before. On the other hand, an unsuccessful result can lead to more emotional heartache and stress, regret, and further surgeries to try to correct the botched job. Because these follow-up surgeries are rarely covered by insurance (especially when the original procedure was deemed cosmetic), the costs will begin to escalate. (And this is absolutely the case when a new surgeon is sought out.)

Although it may be tempting, do not choose your surgeon because his prices are the lowest in town. There may be a reason for this. Similarly, do not assume that a doctor is talented because his fees are high. The Web sites for the American Society of Plastic Surgeons (www.plasticsurgery.org), and the American Society for Aesthetic Plastic Surgery (www.surgery.org), provide national average fee ranges. Different regions of the country have higher or lower prices. Competition for business and a recessive economy has forced many plastic surgeons to offer deep discounts. Research and select the best doctor for your teen's problem. Then discuss fee arrangements.

National Average Costs for Common Teen Procedures

The following table shows average costs for common procedures as reported by the American Society of Plastic Surgeons (ASPS) and the American Society for Aesthetic Plastic Surgery (ASAPS). Note that these are *average* costs, meaning fees can still vary greatly from region to region—and tend to be a lot higher in metropolitan areas. A better way to see if your surgeon's fees are in the ballpark is to compare them with those of other surgeons in your area.

Type of Surgery	Average Cost (ASPS)	Average Cost (ASAPS)
Rhinoplasty	$3,833	$4,493
Otoplasty	$2,549	$3,104
Gynecomastia correction	$3,400	$3,294
Breast reduction	$4,236	$5,634
Chin augmentation	$1,936	$2,269
Fat injections	$1,489	$1,797
Laser hair removal	$503/session/area	$331/session/area
Lower-body lift	$8,073	$7,809
Breast lift	$4,236	$4,414

In addition to value, consider your child's safety. You and your child must be in a comfortable place physically and emotionally to go through the process. Find a doctor who understands your child and the problem. Find a doctor who will stick by you and your child. Your surgeon must have a combination of compassion, understanding, and surgical skill to solve your child's problem. There can be no shortcuts when it comes to surgery. Results are permanent. (Chapter 4 addresses things to keep in mind when choosing your surgeon.)

The Cost of Surgery

In considering the surgeon and his fee, be aware that there are multiple costs involved. The surgeon requires an anesthesiologist, who generates a fee—usually on a per-hour basis. In addition, the surgery must occur in a facility—a hospital, a freestanding surgical center, or an office-based facility—which adds to the total cost.

The following questions are important to ask so that you are aware of all the costs ahead of time.

- Who is assisting with the surgery, and how is that person paid?
- Where will the surgery be done, and what is that cost?
- Who is performing the anesthesia, and what is his cost?
- Where is the recovery, and will there be an additional fee for that facility?
- How often will the surgeon see me? What is the follow-up regimen, and is it included in the price?

Although your insurance company isn't likely to foot the bill for the surgery, there are exceptions. Speak to your plastic surgeon, and find out if the procedure has any chance of being covered. Join forces with your doctor's office to navigate the insurance bureaucracy. Your surgeon's office likely has many patients who desire authorizations, so doing some of the legwork yourself may yield quicker results, if there are any to be had.

> Although your insurance company isn't likely to foot the bill for the surgery, there are exceptions. Speak to your plastic surgeon, and find out if the procedure has any chance of being covered. Join forces with your doctor's office to navigate the insurance bureaucracy.

Insurance Companies: Policies on Coverage

Read the statement below from the medical policy of a major health care insurance company:

> Cosmetic surgery is performed upon normal or abnormal structures for the primary purpose of <u>changing or improving physical appearance</u>.
>
> Reconstructive surgery is performed incidental to an injury, sickness, or congenital anomaly when the primary purpose is to <u>improve physiological functioning</u> of the involved part of the body.

The policy further explained that cosmetic surgery is not covered but reconstructive surgery is. Unfortunately, it's all a word game. What we consider reconstructive quality-of-life surgery may be what they deem cosmetic.

The decision-making process for coverage is often arbitrary and can vary from company to company.

This is indicative of industry standards. If you can hear, you don't need ear surgery, no matter what your ears look like. If you can breathe, plastic surgery on your nose is not covered. Regardless of your breast size, coverage for surgery to change their size is difficult to obtain. Breast asymmetry is not a functional concern—even though this means your teen will have to customize her bras and bathing suits in order to keep them balanced. Restoring normal and balanced anatomy in general is insufficient.

Case in point: A letter from an insurance company to one of my patients, in which the above statement appeared, specifically added that correction of lopsided or prominent ears and breast reduction for males with gynecomastia was excluded from policy coverage.

Insurance companies do not consider psychological liabilities from the altered body part justifiable. So the psychological trauma of a child with prominent ears or asymmetrical breasts does not qualify as sufficient reason to cover the surgery.

Ironically, you can be born without a breast and your insurance will not cover surgery to add one, but if you lose one from a mastectomy, your insurance will likely cover the surgery to replace it. Similarly, some insurance companies will pay for surgery to remove excess skin following weight loss after bariatric surgery (bypass or LAP-BAND) but not for those who lose the weight on their own.

If you are unable to breathe through your nose, insurance companies will consider coverage for rhinoplasty but only for the part that affects your breathing. Anyone who thinks that the mere claim that he has a deviated septum will pay for a nose job is in for a surprise. Those days are long over. An insurance company will want thorough documentation of at least six months of conservative treatment, which basically entails nasal sprays, even though they may be of no benefit or could be harmful. The insurance company may also want you to endure the additional expense of a CAT scan to document what the physician exam already notes.

If your daughter's breasts are oversized, insurance companies have arbitrary requirements on how much needs to be removed before you are considered for reimbursement. Many also stipulate weight requirements for patients, and if they are not met, legitimate complaints of back pain, rashes, and bra-strap discomfort are dismissed. If your child is even slightly overweight, the company may dismiss your claim, requiring that she thin down first. Before considering paying, insurers may ask for six months of conservative therapy with anti-inflammatory medicines, custom bras, physical therapy, and dermatologic care for rashes. Most frustrating is that each company sets its own requirements, and they change frequently—and usually not in your favor.

Attempts at federal legislation to change these insurance policy practices, like the Children's Access to Reconstructive Evaluation and Surgery (CARES) Act, have routinely failed to make it out' of congressional committee.

I have witnessed many heartbreaking instances when insurance companies failed to cover what were clearly important surgeries that would impact a teen's emotional and physical health.

- David was a young adolescent who was horribly teased because of his very prominent ears. From a plastic surgical point of view, his defect was a congenital anomaly. The cartilages of his ears were not normal and were a result of a failure of development

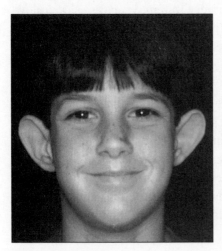 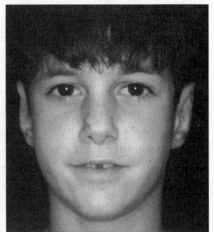

of the anatomical folds prior to birth. A letter and photograph were sent to his insurance company along with supportive letters from his school and pediatrician. The insurance company's response?

> "Our consultant has reviewed all of the supporting information and the following determination has been made: the contract excludes cosmetic procedures. Based on the information provided, it has been determined that the procedure is cosmetic. There are no benefits for this proposed service."

- Ellen was a teenage girl who had matured with significantly asymmetrical breasts. One had essentially failed to develop while the other was large and disfigured. She was so distressed by this that she developed psychological problems and irritable bowel syndrome requiring medication. Her family requested surgical coverage. The insurance company's response?

> "We reviewed the information provided, and our medical team has concluded that it is cosmetic in nature and therefore not covered. . . . New York State's mandate for breast reconstruction applies only to women who have had mastectomies. Therefore, medical necessity has not been demonstrated and services are not certified."

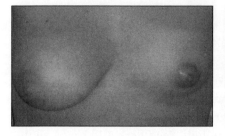 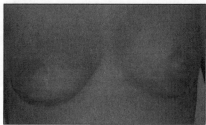

- Joan was an 18-year-old girl who was significantly overweight. She finally took control of her life; through an organized weight-loss program, she reduced herself from 312 pounds to 165 pounds. As a result, she was left with a tremendous amount of hanging skin. She needed a redraping surgery to remove all the excess skin. "I want this more than anything," she said. "I feel so uncomfortable with myself that I hate living in my own skin." Her parents sought coverage for the surgery. The insurance company's response?

  "We have sent your request to a utilization review agency that performs the management functions for your health plan. After reviewing the information our physician reviewer has denied the request."

  Even though she met the criteria proposed by the company—more than six months with the weight off, chronic skin irritations, and hanging skin over the pubic area (demonstrated by a photo)—the procedure was deemed cosmetic. After three appeals, she was finally approved, but the whole process took almost one year!

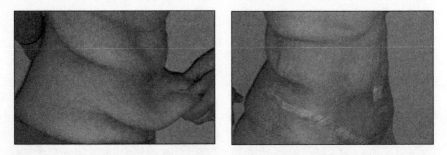

The insurance arena is not fully vested in quality of patient care. As a for-profit business, it is the bottom line, not empathy, that drives it. Decades ago, coverage decisions were made based on letters from physicians—and that was justification enough. Fees were paid based on the operative reports describing complexity of the procedure. Today, everything is computerized and done by codes. Everything has to fit within these codes for coverage. Many insurance companies lump parts of operations together into an unrealistic global fee, thereby allowing them to pay a reduced fee for the services. Some insurance companies further reduce their payments by establishing physician profiles and paying some doctors more or less than others based on this predetermined information. Insurance companies also have negotiators to try and reduce approved fees once the procedure is complete but before payment is rendered. If you select a surgeon who is not within your insurance provider's network, the company may not cover your hospital fees even if the hospital was within the network. These are all moves to reimburse the patient and physician as little as possible and increase the insurance company's profitability.

Tips for Paying for Surgery

The squeaky wheel sometimes does get the grease when dealing with insurance. If you are persistent and keep plugging away with requests and documentations, it can pay off. Some families have successfully taken their case to their government representative to put pressure on the insurance company. Other times, you are up against a brick wall. I have repaired lacerations in my office operating room, and the insurance claims were denied because the service was not performed in a hospital emergency room, even though the overall cost was cheaper to them.

> The squeaky wheel sometimes does get the grease when dealing with insurance. If you are persistent and keep plugging away with requests and documentations, it can pay off.

Because most insurance won't cover plastic surgery, there are other avenues that have opened up to create affordability:

- Some plastic surgeons will offer to do your child's surgery in their offices and may use a CRNA (certified registered nurse anesthetist), which can be less expensive than an MD anesthesiologist. After surgery, their patients may either go home accompanied by a hired nurse or stay overnight in a hotel with a nurse (if they have traveled a distance for their procedure or are not comfortable being home that first night). Although seemingly cheaper, this adds up. Ask your surgeon about other options such as having the surgery in a hospital and staying overnight there if needed. Many hospitals are in competition for the discretionary dollars generated from cosmetic surgery and therefore offer competitive pricing for anesthesia, the facility, and even overnight services. This may turn out to be more cost effective as well as providing more emotional security to your child.

- Consider cutting back on other expenses. Eliminating a vacation that will soon be forgotten may be worth it if it means being able to afford a lifelong change for your child. Keep in mind that if you look at the price of the surgery over the decades of your son or daughter's life, the procedure most likely comes to less than a few dollars a day.

- Very few plastic surgery offices offer independent financing, but companies such as CareCredit (www.carecredit.com), which is endorsed by the American Society of Plastic Surgeons, offer financing to families seeking plastic surgery. By logging on to CareCredit's Web site, you can obtain specifics about individual procedures and terms.

The Bottom Line

The bottom line is that you can't count on insurance to cover even the most basic plastic surgery procedures for teens, even if many doctors would consider them medically necessary. This means that as parents, you will have to decide whether or not a major financial investment in your child's psychological and social well-being is worth the expense. In my experience, parents who weigh the cost versus the value usually find that when the need is defined and agreed upon by both teens and parents and the procedures are done properly with realistic expectations, the investment pays lifelong positive emotional dividends.

The Lowdown on Insurance

Carefully review your insurance policy. Many people think they have better coverage than they do. The cheaper the policy, the less you will be getting in return. Also keep the following points in mind:

1. Just because we (doctor, patient, and family) see the need does not mean that insurance will pay. Insurance is primarily concerned with the bottom line.
2. Most insurance companies require a preauthorization, and their first response is to deny. (That is generally their second and third responses, too.)
3. Be prepared to file an appeal and then reappeal to an outside board. Sometimes these appeals, with careful documentation of necessity, can be resolved in your favor.
4. Make sure you have thorough documentation to build your case. The following table shows the requirements you may need to meet to prove the procedure qualifies for coverage.

Type of Surgery	Your Requirements
Nose surgery	At least six months of conservative treatment CAT scans documenting a deviated septum
Breast reduction	Six months of conservative care, custom bra, physical therapy, and anti-inflammatory medications Close to ideal body weight Dermatologist documentation of rashes Orthopedist documentation of back pain
Weight-loss surgery	Proof that hanging skin is hampering function

5. Take personal responsibility (rather than depending on the doctor's office) for challenging the insurance company decision if it comes back unfavorable.
6. Obtain approvals in writing.

83

PART TWO

PROCEDURES

6

Introduction
to Procedures

P ART TWO LOOKS AT THE DETAILS, including the risks, of the most common plastic surgical solutions for teens. Each chapter following this one discusses physical problems that can cause psychosocial distress and offers surgical solutions to those problems. I take you through the process of evaluating an affected teen in the initial consultation and moving through the surgical evaluation and treatment to recovery and the quality-of-life enhancements that follow. These chapters include personal attestations of parents and teens about their feelings in coping with these physical problems and the relief following their correction. These testimonials are not advertisements for my own practice but are included so that the reader can get into the heads and hearts of people facing a similar problem.

This introduction takes you through the process of using the services of a plastic surgeon. As you read through these overviews, keep in mind that what you experience may vary from the basic template I describe.

Before you begin the steps, remember that the most important thing is to be armed with as much information as possible and to be in touch with your teen's psychological and emotional (as well as physical) well-being.

The Initial Phone Call

That first call to the first office is where the process truly begins. For most, the call means entering the unknown, and parents are nervous about making it. How the call is received can make all the difference. The receptionists are the gatekeepers to the office. They signal what is ahead. Be aware of the impression these individuals make. Are they friendly and welcoming? Will they accommodate your teen's schedule? Are they answering your questions? Do you get the impression that the office will be looking forward to your visit? (For more on how to best handle this call as well as the consultation itself, see the checklists in chapter 4.)

The Consultation

There are many ways to perform certain surgical procedures. Surgeons develop their own style and have their own aesthetic. It is in the consultation that you make sure that the surgeon's ideas are in keeping with what you are looking for.

The consultation can be intimidating for your teen. He or she could be embarrassed about openly discussing their problem, especially if it involves a sensitive area like breasts or has been a source of ridicule. How the surgeon handles your teen's discomfort will be very informative about what you can expect from the surgeon later.

To prepare for my consultations, I like to send out the patient information package in advance of the appointment. This allows the teen and family to fill out their demographics and answer the medical questions thoroughly and completely in privacy and at their own pace. It prevents delays and backups in the office when they arrive with all the "chart" information prepared. It also shows commitment on their part to having a meaningful and mutual consultation.

Once the patient has arrived at the office, I like to have my staff introduce themselves prior to any physical examination. This breaks down the barriers and helps to create a friendlier atmosphere. I have my nurse escort the parents and teen into a room, where I will come to introduce myself and get background on the purpose of the visit. This usually entails conversations about the teen and his or her life. I like to get a feel for the child and observe the family interaction as they respond to my questions. Once the lines of communication are established, we can be more relaxed in addressing the problem.

If the problem is facial, then there is usually less embarrassment, and with the aid of photography and computer imaging, the teen, parents, and surgeon can look at the issues together. The morphing program allows for discussion on what can and cannot be done (this process is discussed in greater detail in chapter 7). The archival program allows the patient to see before-and-after examples of other patients and how the results compared to the morphed proposals.

If the problem is in the breast area, then it is imperative that a nurse and the teen's family (unless directed otherwise) be in the room for the physical exam. The mere fact that a stranger is touching your teen's breast can be overwhelming, and the surgeon needs to handle this very sensitively. I discuss the process thoroughly before the exam, which reduces a teen's feeling of vulnerability as much as possible. I make the initial observation brief. After the first exam is complete and we've had further discussion, it is usually easier to reexamine and go into more detail about the particular issue. Sometimes it is better to limit the exam and offer the patient and family a second visit where they feel more comfortable reentering a familiar environment.

I insist that my patients have more than one visit to my office. I want to double-check everything, including the family dynamic. The more we get to know each other, the easier the process becomes.

Medical Photography

Plastic surgery is a very visual specialty, and therefore before-and-after photography is essential to the record-keeping process. Having photos made can be intimidating to young patients, especially when it involves the breasts or other private areas. Many offices send patients to professional studios to have the photos made—I am totally against this. I take all my own photographs in the security of the office. That way, the patient maintains privacy and feels less vulnerable in exposing an already-troubling area. Digital photography allows us to keep an archive of the patient's record. Archives can be helpful in discussing the patient's progress, and they come in handy when we need to print copies for family members who may not have been present at the follow-up.

The Pre-op Visit

I believe it is imperative to reevaluate all surgical candidates as we come closer to the time for surgery. Many times, the interval between initial consultation and surgery can be long, especially when we're working around a teen's busy schedule. Sometimes things change—weight, attitudes, family dynamics. It is good to reconnect.

The pre-op appointment is where I revisit my operative plan. Many of our procedures require ink "markings," or visual landmarks for the surgery. Some surgeons do these the day of surgery in the admitting area. I do not. I see my patients in my office a few days in advance, and I make all the marks in the privacy of the office with an indelible ink, which will be removed after surgery. This reinforces my work plan and provides me with comfort in knowing that my plan will work. It also allows the patient to see the proposed incision lines and live with them at home. In addition, it allows for the day of surgery to proceed more smoothly. The teen and family are nervous, and the hours before surgery are no time to begin a "mark out." I would rather use that time to say hello, provide assurances, check my marks, review the plan, and get to work.

At the pre-op visit, I give appropriate prescriptions for antibiotics and control of postoperative pain and nausea. With elective plastic surgery, pain should diminish rapidly. I always tell my patients that if they are experiencing significant pain after the procedure, I want to see them to rule out a problem.

The Operating Room

Surgeons can forget that, although the operating room is familiar turf to them, it is terrifying to a patient. It is sterile and filled with strange machines and unfamiliar people. It is beneficial to have a family member accompany teen patients into the operating room and be with them as they enter anesthesia. I also make sure that I am by his or her side as the teen goes to sleep. By now, the patient trusts me, and it can ease his or her nervousness to see a familiar face. I want my patient to see me last before going to sleep and see me first upon waking up.

The Recovery Room and Follow-up

It is important to have the family reunited as soon after the surgery as possible. I like to move the patient to the recovery room, brief the family, and then bring the family into the recovery room as quickly as possible. I stay in the recovery area until the teen is fully awake and comfortable. This assures family of my total commitment.

Once the patient is discharged and sent home, I ask the family to call the office to let us know they have arrived home safely and to give us updated phone contacts, if needed. The office will call later that day to check on them again, and I will call in the evening to answer any questions that have come up.

Different surgeons have different policies on who sees the patient and how often during recovery. I am a hands-on surgeon. I see my early post-op patients often and examine and change their bandages myself. I see teens frequently throughout the first year as they heal. After that, I see them at least yearly as physical maturity progresses. My door is always open for a teen for any concerns.

7

The Ears:
The Frame of the Face

I was made fun of at school
They called me a fool.
But that all changed
When my ears were rearranged.

—GENEVIEVE, Age 16

FINGERTIP FACTS

☞ Ear deformities are either congenital or traumatic.

☞ They can range from minor earlobe problems to complete ear absence.

☞ The ear is fully developed by age 6.

☞ Structural ear problems manifest early in life.

☞ Social implications can be significant, so surgery should be considered early.

THIS CHAPTER IS SPECIAL in that it deals with issues that have strong social implications occurring much earlier than the teen years. Although there is a spectrum that defines ears from the typical to the atypical to the truly deformed, structural ear problems in a young child can be distressing to new parents. Approximately 5 percent of the population has some kind of ear abnormality that falls outside the range of ethnic variability and cultural acceptance.

Ears develop during the sixth to twelfth week of intrauterine life and are adult size by age 6. At birth, it is clear whether or not a child has normal or abnormal ears.

A child can be born without an ear on one or both sides. This condition is called microtia and can occur as an isolated deformity or as part of a number of congenital problems, including hearing loss. Reconstructions are complicated and require the skill of dedicated specialists. Less severe but obvious problems include ears with very little structural support (cryptotia) as well as very large ears (macrotia). Children with these conditions have normal hearing but still require complex reconstructions. Ideally, parents of these children are referred to a plastic surgical specialist for a treatment plan early in the child's life.

There are still other ear abnormalities that are far less severe, and parents of an affected child may hope their child will grow into them or live with them. One such abnormality is the prominent ear—casually and cruelly called "jug ears," "Dumbo ears," and "Mickey Mouse ears." These are ears that protrude far beyond the side of the head and result from a failure of the embryonic cartilage to fold back.

Even though prominent ears can be a source of tremendous teasing and angst in a socially vulnerable child, many people and most insurance companies view this failure of folding to be a cosmetic issue. Parents often seek out plastic surgical help only when their child becomes significantly tormented.

There can also be many variations on the shape of earlobes and the shape of the rims of the ears. Some lobes are large, and some barely existent. Some ears have excess cartilage points and have been referred to as "Mr. Spock ears" (in reference to the *Star Trek* character).

Problems with ears can be one-sided or involve both, and it's not uncommon for one ear to be different from the other.

This is not a text on ear reconstruction but rather a look at common ear deformities in children. This chapter focuses on the following problems:

- Prominent ears
- Excess cartilage
- Ear trauma, including cauliflower ear and problems from piercings—stretched and torn lobes, ear infections, and keloids (extreme scarring)

The Prominent Ear Deformity: 'Don't Call Me Dumbo!'

Prominent ears are by far the most common and distressing aesthetic problem to the preteen population. This involves incomplete folding of the ears so that they don't sit close to the head. As noted earlier, ears are essentially fully grown by age 6, and what you see is what you have. Taping, gluing, or merely hoping to grow into them are often efforts in vain. In 2008, more than 8,000 children between 13 and 19 underwent surgical correction of prominent ears. This procedure made up nearly 30 percent of surgeries for this age group, ranking third behind rhinoplasty and breast reduction. The numbers are even greater when younger individuals are considered.

Why is this problem so important? This is often the first body-image issue a young child faces. As soon as socialization occurs, the possibility of derisive comments exists. An emotionally healthy child leaving the security of home to interact in school may discover that the world can be a cruel place. The relentless comments of peers who delight in ridicule can break the spirit of a developing ego. You can only be called "Dumbo," "Mickey Mouse," or "Jughead" so many times before social isolation occurs.

It is usually these negative emotional experiences that ultimately bring the child to the plastic surgeon. Fortunately, the usual time of emotional anxiety over protruding ears coincides with the structural maturity of the ears, therefore allowing for early correction and abatement of the psychological abuse.

Considering Surgery for Prominent Ears: Proaction Is the Best Reaction

If your child has structural ear issues and you notice behavioral changes in him or her, such as unwillingness to socialize or refusal to wear short hairstyles, be proactive and discuss the possibility of surgical correction.

Ignoring the problem or trying to soothe the child rarely has a lasting benefit. Surgery may not be for every child, but the evaluation and discussion is well worth it.

I have seen children in my office as young as 5 begging for the surgery. They would jump onto the operating table in a flash if given the chance. I have also seen children who were glad to know of the possibility for correction but were not ready, in spite of parental prodding. Young minds know what is going on, and it is best to include them in the discussion and observe their reactions. Timing should be when the child is ready.

In my experience, most children who have felt the burden of ridicule welcome the opportunity to have the problem fixed. They know from looking at their classmates—and from those classmates telling them as much—that their ears are different. Parents are also grateful to find out about the options for surgery. Many times, pediatricians, who may be the first to hear about the child's distress, encourage parents to seek plastic surgical consultation.

Demonstrating the proposed improvement from surgical correction of the prominent ear is easy and straightforward. Because the majority of problems stem from an absence of the major fold of the ear—the ante-helical fold—the simple folding back of the ear basically shows the prospective patient what can be done. Computer imaging of the ears also helps children and their parents visualize the change. It is this glimpse at having ears like their peers that usually solidifies the decision to go forward with surgery.

At this point, it behooves parents to question the plastic surgeon about his experience in performing an otoplasty—surgical correction of prominent ears. Although many surgeons are taught this procedure, there is a steep learning curve to creating a natural-looking ear. It is best to find that surgeon who is adept at ear reconstructions. Many pediatric plastic surgeons have developed strong skill sets in the entire range of ear deformities and can best plan for your child's surgery. Ask to see many before-and-after pictures, and ask if you can speak with families of children who have undergone the procedure.

Are you and your child ready for surgery? The following are green-light and red-flag indicators that can help you decide.

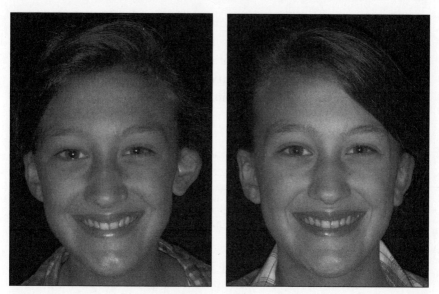

A 12-year-old girl with a one-sided prominent ear deformity. It was corrected with an otoplasty to match the "normal" side.

Green Lights

- Your child is distressed over the shape of his or her ears, and it is affecting daily living.
- Your child is willing to undergo a surgical procedure and comply with the recovery.
- You understand that insurance is unlikely to pay for the procedure.
- You are secure with the chosen surgeon.

Red Flags

- Your child is not ready for surgery; you are pushing to go forward with it.
- Your child is not ready to be compliant with the time involved in recovery.
- You expect insurance to pay for it.

I try to gain the confidence of young people by asking them to draw me a picture of what their ears look like and how other people see them. The drawings often come as a surprise to parents, who may have never comprehended the depth of the anxiety. Often parents are even more surprised when they see their child's postsurgery drawings and how their view of self has improved.

> Life before surgery was difficult with ears that stuck out like Dumbo; which is what I was called. Let's just say that when your ears literally stuck straight out from your head, it gives other children plenty of chances to make fun of you.
>
> After years of coming home from school in tears, my parents decided to look into correction.
>
> When the procedure was over I remember going from "Sad Scott to Glad Scott." I remember going to school like there was never a problem.
>
> Even to this day, when I look back at all the unhappy pictures I well up; then think about all the happy pictures in my future: graduation, prom, vacations and parties.

These drawings are a typical example of how children use non-verbal communication to express feelings of dismay over a perceived deformity and elation after surgical correction.

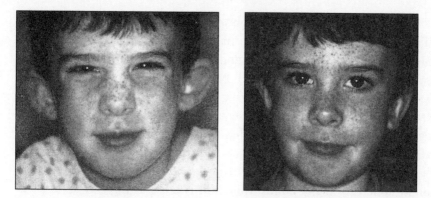

A prominent ear deformity in a 6-year old boy, shown before surgery and then immediately after surgical correction.

> Having surgery was the best thing I ever did. It raised my self-esteem and made e feel more comfortable. It changed me!
> —Scott, age 19*

* See Scott's drawings in Chapter14.

Scott, years later.

Before the Surgery: What to Expect

It is a big step to go from the theoretical idea of having your young child's ears corrected to the actual surgery. Before the procedure can be planned, parents need to know what to expect. They must be informed that all surgery carries risks such as bleeding and infection, although with otoplasty, it is very low. Most often, if there is a problem, it is the failure to create identical ears. On rare occasions, an ear "pops back out" because of broken stitches. This would necessitate a revisional surgery at a future date.

Because most patients are young, general anesthesia is the norm. (Teens, who can understand the surgical process and cooperate, could have the surgery with sedation and local anesthesia.) The procedure is ambulatory, and your child will be going home once fully recovered from anesthesia. There is often a big, fluffy bandage protecting the ears. Remarkably, there is little pain associated with ear surgery, and oral analgesic medications are not needed after a day or two. Some surgeons will, at the time of surgery, inject a long-acting local anesthetic to further assist in patient comfort. By the time the surgeon makes the evening phone call to the family, the child is often at the computer or in front of the television.

Next is the follow-up visit. I like to see the patient forty-eight to seventy-two hours after surgery to change the bandage. Parents need to know that their child will be home for about a week to rest and allow the surgical sites to heal. At the end of that week, the bandage is replaced with a headband that goes over the ears to protect them for another three weeks. Patients and their parents must realize that the recovery process involves abstaining from sports for one month.

> Over the past few years, I have become increasingly concerned about the appearance of my ears. It wasn't that my ears had suddenly changed but rather that I had come to realize just how much they protruded. I became constantly worried that others would see them and ridicule me.
>
> I did the only thing I knew that I could—hid them by growing my hair very long. Sometimes they were still visible. I was miserable and felt as if I was prevented from doing things because of my preoccupation with my misshapen ears.
>
> Since the otoplasty (ear pinning), I no longer have ears that bother me. They look normal. I feel like a new person. I am more confident and have a great sense of relief and freedom.
>
> I am now able to concentrate on successfully completing my senior year in high school and make plans for college without the worry of how I looked.
> —Karen, age 17

The Surgery: Otoplasty

Otoplasty requires two basic steps: a re-creation of the absent ante-helical fold and, if necessary, a reduction in the depth of the bowl of the ear, the concha. (See figure 7.1.)

The incisions for this procedure are most often made behind the ear, placing the scar inconspicuously in a fold. The cartilage can be reduced and folded with stitches that secure the position of the ear until healing has rendered the result permanent. The skin is closed with dissolving sutures, thereby avoiding the anxiety of having to move the newly shaped ears.

The surgery, in experienced hands, takes about ninety minutes. Within two to three hours after the surgery, most children are ready to go home. My personal criteria for releasing a patient are that the patient be pain free and without nausea, able to tolerate food, and able to walk and go to the bathroom. These indicators reinforce to parents that their child is truly ready for discharge.

A phone call to the family later in the day to answer any questions further ensures that my role in their child's recovery did not end in the recovery room.

Otoplasty at an early age can eliminate years of emotional distress and obviate sad situations I have encountered, like that of a teen who would Krazy Glue her ears to her head before going on dates so she would look normal for the evening.

A WORD OF CAUTION: **Otoplasty must be performed by an experienced surgeon.** In the wrong hands complications can go beyond simply needing to redo the operation. There can be irreparable damage to the shape of the ears ranging from overcorrection, producing the so-called "telephone ear," where it is virtually plastered to the side of the head, to so much cartilage removed that the ear canal narrows, causing pain. I once saw a teen whose canals were so narrowed because of scarring that he could not even put an iPod earbud in his ear.

Excess Cartilage: 'I'm Not Spock'

There are variants of cartilage deformities in ears that, although minor in comparison to some, still create significant consternation, especially in this era of short hairstyles. Gone are the Beatles cuts that hid a lot of flaws.

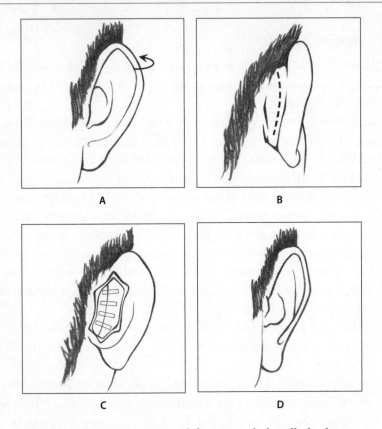

Figure 7.1 (A) a prominent ear deformity with the telltale absent ante-helical fold; (B) the typical incision pattern on the back of the ear to access the cartilage, fold it, and bring the ear back into a normal position; (C) the placement of stitches to fold the ear cartilage; (D) the normal ear architecture after the folding of the ear cartilage.

Darwinian tubercles (named for Charles Darwin, who was the first to publish a description of them) are overgrowths of cartilage on the middle and/or upper parts of the rim of the ear. They are present in about 10 percent of the population. Socially conscious teens often want them gone, and they can be removed under local anesthesia with little downtime.

Ear Trauma: 'Damage Control'

Another major category of ear deformities results from trauma. Repeated trauma to the cartilages can cause the ear to lose its shape, producing a "cauliflower" ear. When teens have their ears pierced, it can lead to stretching, tearing, keloids, and infections.

I wanted plastic surgery because of the appearance of one of my ears. Although once a symbol of my high school greatness as a wrestler, it now was a source of attention I no longer wanted. Most people did not understand that this "cauliflower deformity" resulted from rigorous training on the mat without proper protective headgear. I grew tired of explaining why my ears were different.

Since the surgery (multiple small procedures) to reestablish the folds in my ear, I feel that my appearance has improved as well as my self confidence.

—Jeff, age 19

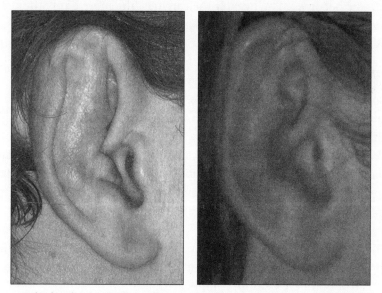

As a high school wrestler, Jeff experienced a "cauliflower" ear deformity from repeated ear trauma. Multiple small surgical procedures were needed to re carve out "normal" ear anatomy. The lesson is for athletes to use protective head gear to avoid the problem

The Cauliflower Ear Deformity

Repeated trauma to the ear, as can occur in contact sports like wrestling, may result in the ear losing much of its normal architecture. When the delicate folds of the ear are lost, the deformity is called a "cauliflower" ear. It is prevented by encouraging young athletes to wear protective headgear. For many, it seems that these injuries sustained on the "field of battle" are "badges of courage." Unfortunately, long after the glory days are gone, the deformity remains and is difficult to fully correct.

Surgery to improve a cauliflower ear requires many small outpatient procedures to essentially recarve ear anatomy into the amorphous blocks of cartilage swollen by repeated trauma. An "ounce of prevention" with headgear is worth "a pound of cure."

Problems from Piercings

In some societies, stretched-out earlobes are accepted. Our society is not one of these. The problem is that many kids today want multiple ear piercings—and not just in the lobes. The more holes, the weaker the tissue becomes. The heavier the earrings, the more likely the risk of stretching and tearing, as the holes become larger and larger.

When the damage is from torn or stretched lobes, the plastic surgical solution is to close the holes and reshape the earlobe. The lobes can then be safely repierced in about six weeks. In many cases, only one earlobe has stretched or torn. This is presumably caused by pressure from the telephone, and perhaps in the new era of text messaging, this problem will become less common.

When discs are used instead of earrings, the holes can be very large. Repair requires a more complicated shifting of tissues to reconstruct a normal-appearing lobe. But, parents, take heart when you see these piercings: Even the largest of lobe holes can be fixed!

Piercings through the cartilage, however, are a different story. Cartilage has a poor blood supply, which makes healing potentially slow and increases the risk of infection and possibly ear rim collapse. Reconstruction here is more complicated.

Even if the ears aren't torn or stretched, piercings can cause problems. Many youngsters get their ears pierced and don't take care of the sites. Earrings can become imbedded in swollen and tender lobes. Treatment requires removal of the earrings, often with a local anesthetic block to control the pain.

Keloids

Keloids are thickened and overdeveloped scars that are larger than the original site of trauma. They result from an overproduction of collagen, the basic building block of healing. Ear keloids are most often seen on the lobes at the site of a piercing. They occur most frequently in the black population. The scar tissue can grow to be quite large and look like a grape on the ear.

Treatment is difficult because of the recurrent nature of the heavy scarring. Often the area requires pretreatment with a series of steroid injections to soften the keloid scar. This is then followed by surgical excision and reconstruction. In very difficult cases that continue to recur, very low-dose radiation therapy is added to the immediate postoperative regimen. The radiation can slow the collagen growth and prevent new keloid formation. Although safe, it is only used when all other

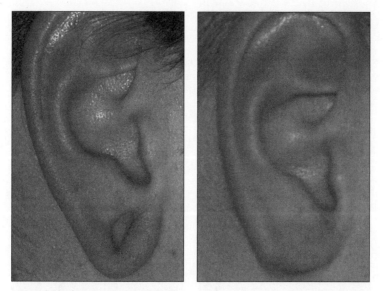

Large hole from piercing with discs. After earlobe reconstruction to close the hole and reestablish normal ear shape.

treatments fail, and it is part of a complete program with steroids and surgery.

A WORD OF CAUTION: Individuals who develop keloids need a warning to avoid repiercing to prevent recurrences. If the patient wants to wear earrings, he or she must use only clip-ons.

If you or your teen suspects a problem arising from trauma to the ears, it is best to act early. First, stop the problem: wear protective headgear in contact sports and remove earrings if the ears are inflamed or hurt. If you suspect a keloid forming, seek professional help early to try and stop its progression.

Final Thoughts

Correction of ear deformities is one of the most rewarding interventions a pediatric plastic surgeon can conduct. The results are immediate and last a lifetime.

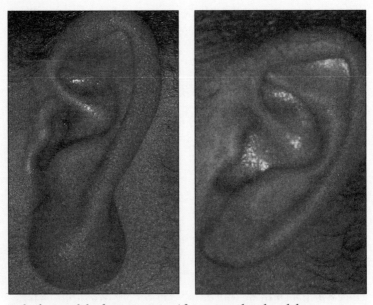

Keloid on earlobe from piercing. After removal and earlobe reconstruction.

Tormented children have found peace. They're carefree with their hairstyles, no longer afraid to let their ears show. Because ears are fully developed so early in childhood, we can put affected children on a happy path before psychological damage overwhelms them. Every postsurgery photograph I take shows a big smile, and every visit ends with a thank you from the parents and child.

8

The Face:
Finding the Balance

"I am happy people find me attractive,
but it is really a matter of mathematics."

—PAULINA PORIZKOVA, supermodel

FINGERTIP FACTS

☞ Rhinoplasty (nose job) is the most common procedure performed on teens.

☞ When a skilled plastic surgeon looks at the nose, the entire face
is evaluated.

☞ Balance and proportion create facial beauty: The whole is often
greater than the sum of the parts.

☞ Computer imaging can be helpful in visualizing an outcome.

I F YOU ASK PEOPLE to identify a single procedure that is practically
synonymous with plastic surgery, they will say rhinoplasty—more
commonly known as "the nose job." And indeed it is one of the old-
est procedures on record, dating back to the sixteenth century, when
noses were reconstructed by Turkish surgeons during the Ottoman

wars. Many parents today can recall their own teenage years, when fellow classmates got the "rite of passage" nose job at age 16 during the spring break.

In 2009, more than 40,000 rhinoplasties were performed on teenagers and another 80,000 on people aged 20 to 29. And these statistics reflect only procedures performed by board-certified plastic surgeons. If we include procedures done by Ear, Nose, and Throat surgeons, the numbers increase. This is a very popular and common procedure and one that has been a canon of plastic surgery for many years.

As a young girl my daughter had an adorable, well-proportioned face. During her adolescent years she developed a bump on her nose and her chin seemed to recede.

She was teased in school and out. Her self-esteem plummeted. She hid her face behind long hair, and her eyes rarely lifted off the floor. She would cry frequently. I could see that she was desperately unhappy.

I told her she was beautiful inside and out; but that didn't begin to take the edge off of her misery. Finally we talked about "options," when and if she was ever ready.

Shortly before we were to move to another town and school district she came to my husband and me and asked for surgery. She wanted a fresh start. She was now almost 16.

Alana needed to have her face made more harmonious. She needed not only nose surgery but chin surgery also. This was done as a combination procedure with an oral-maxillofacial surgeon advancing the chin and a plastic surgeon refining her nose.

The surgery went very well, and as the swelling was decreasing we could see her happiness increasing. Her self-esteem quickly rose. She tried out for cheerleading at her new school and her social life was full.

Alana began to take an interest in her appearance and became outgoing. She could now look people in the eye. We all agree that the facial balancing was a life altering experience.

She is now 26 and works in the fashion industry.

—Laura (mother)

Today, we not only have advances in surgical techniques but a greater understanding of what constitutes a beautiful face. Any serious information a surgeon imparts to teens and families about nasal surgery must also include information about facial balance—the relationship of the nose to the rest of the face, primarily the chin and the cheeks.

In this chapter, I discuss the nose, the chin, and the cheeks individually and also collectively as they relate to facial balance. I give a thorough explanation of surgical techniques and new advances in the field, taking into consideration the potential special needs of your teen. Let's start with the basics.

Today, we not only have advances in surgical techniques but a greater understanding of what constitutes a beautiful face. Any serious information a surgeon imparts to teens and families about nasal surgery must also include information about facial balance—the relationship of the nose to the rest of the face, primarily the chin and the cheeks.

How the Face Grows

Puberty and its resultant growth spurts—both the physical and emotional components—can be surprising to teens and parents. Height increases, breasts develop (hopefully only in girls), and faces change. Suddenly the amorphous faces of childhood begin to take on distinct characteristics, and familial traits appear. Infants and small children have round faces with ill-defined noses and chins and chubby cheeks. With the eruption of teeth, the face begins to change, and it continues to change with each stage of dental development. As all the teeth move into place, the front of the face responds to these driving forces. Small button noses with little bones and cartilages begin to grow, and as the nose pushes out, the upper and lower jaws begin to take on their adult shape. Orthodontic studies have shown that 90 percent of nasal growth occurs between the ages of 13 and14. Puberty and hormonal changes further complete facial shape and cause skin changes like sweat gland formation and facial hair in boys. The once angelic faces of childhood can morph into new and unfamiliar landscapes.

This rapid change in physical appearance can bring either joy or distress to your teen. It is important to be supportive through this transformation, which seems almost revolutionary to the anxious adolescent. Part of this support is allowing your teen to express his or her feelings about his or her appearance openly and honestly without judgment.

What teens are instinctively responding to is a change in the balance of their face. It has been known for centuries and across cultures that balance and harmony are synonymous with beauty. The Greeks were obsessed with symmetry, and Renaissance Italians like Leonardo da Vinci called it the "Golden Mean." Music and art from Michelangelo to Mozart and architecture from the pyramids to the Parthenon have been appreciated as perfect and all fell into the Divine proportions.

If there is an alteration in the traditional balance of the face at puberty, teens may not always be able to identify exactly what is bothering them, and sometimes they may even focus on the wrong anatomical part, but they know something is askew. This is a delicate time but one in which concerned parents can help the teen redefine an image that he or she will project happily and comfortably for the rest of his or her life.

The face cannot be hidden. It is visible for all to see and judge. Beauty may allegedly be in the eye of the beholder, but we have to acknowledge that we live in a society that is increasingly focused on appearance. I have had many teens in my office confiding in tears that they've been called "Pinocchio," "Toucan," or "Parrot Beak."

Considering Surgery

A plastic surgical consultation can help settle teen angst by discussing what is possible and what is not possible, and the appropriate timings. Knowledge is empowering, and young minds are very receptive to helpful information.

Whereas anxious teens just know they are unhappy with their looks, skilled plastic surgeons with knowledge of facial balance can quantify and objectify those distressed feelings. Taking lessons from both science and art, we understand that perceived beauty falls into ratios and proportions. We do not need to become bogged down with trying to give every face a width that is two-thirds its length or make structures fall into the ratio of phi (1.618:1), but the numbers do give us reference points to help individuals understand their issues and help us achieve surgical satisfaction. (See figure 8.1.)

Digital photography and computer imaging software allow a teen to see the changes that are possible. The patient and family can see together, with the surgeon, the entire face in multiple views. The surgeon can then introduce proposed changes to the graphic image to balance the face. He could make adjustments to the nose, the chin, the cheeks, or any combination of these.

The following sections look at what constitutes facial harmony and the variations that could be causing stress to your teen and preventing them from developing a healthy body image.

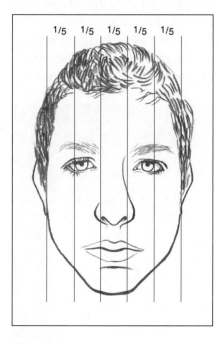

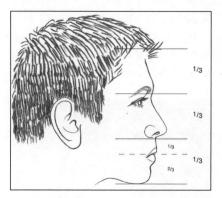

Figure 8.1 These illustrations define the ideal mathematical proportions of the face. They are known as the "divine proportions" or the "Golden Mean," for balance and harmony.

'It's as Plain as the Nose on Your Face'

A nose that is well balanced seems to blend into the rest of the face and add to overall attractiveness. A nose that is out of sync with the rest of the face can be a source of great distress and negatively affect self-esteem. It cannot be hidden or camouflaged and may begin to occupy a majority of a teen's mental energy and focus.

If a nose is too long, too short, too thick, too droopy, or too upturned, there are techniques to correct these disproportions. The patient and family will, of course, have certain anxieties about reconstructing the nose. A parent's anxiety may relate to their own experience of having a nose surgery as a teen or knowing someone who did. Memories or stories of being awake and hearing bones break may still linger. Surgery in the past was imprecise and unpredictable, and thoughts of the "one style fits all" nose may hinder some from seeking a consultation.

Today, rhinoplasty is very sophisticated. It has evolved far beyond large bump removal and turned-up tips. Each feature of the nose can be refined. We can analyze and address each aspect of the nose so that we

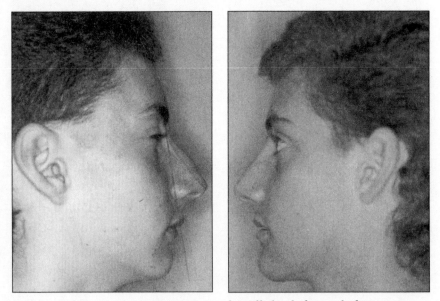

A 16-year-old boy with prominent nose and small chin before and after surgery. Facial balancing procedure with rhinoplasty and chin augmentation. (Note the lines to establish ideal facial proportions on before photo.)

can have results that look natural and are harmonious with the other facial features.

A WORD OF CAUTION: Keep in mind that this is structural surgery, and the changes are permanent. It is paramount that you know that your teen is having the surgery for him or herself and not to please you or because of peer pressures.

Having been raised in New York City I was keenly aware of the importance society places on beauty. I resented this type of judgment because it deflected from meaningful values. I was going to raise my children so they did not place such a high value on external modifiers. Then reality set in. By the time my daughter was 11 years old her nose became the prominent feature on her face. It became the target of cruel and mean spirited comments by her "peers." My high-leveled intentions were replaced with anxiety as I saw my daughter's self-esteem being worn down bit by bit, day by day.

Over the next year, in spite of parental protection, it became clear that we were heading into psychological deep water. We needed help. Plastic surgery on her nose would not be to make her more "beautiful." She was only 12 and had years of growth and development ahead of her. It was to stop the continual blows to her ego, constantly assaulting her self-esteem. The procedure would be very limited—just to refine the bump—nothing that would affect facial growth. Our family made a decision to help her, knowing that with growth, future revision might be needed.

The surgery turned out to be invaluable. She felt good about herself as if a burden had been lifted. It allowed her to concentrate on other things besides her looks. Interestingly, as she grew over the years she did regain part of her "bump," but she did not care. Her ego had become solid. The surgery was performed for a specific reason at a critical time, and I believe that had it not been done, the consequences would have been devastating to her self-esteem, and things would have been different for her.

—Barbara (mother)

Timing

Teens are usually in a hurry to have their procedures done, yet they have very busy lives. There are two important timing issues to consider. First is the age appropriateness for the surgery, second is when can it fit into a teen's schedule.

We know that nasal growth is in its final phases on average between 13 and 14 years of age. Pediatric plastic surgeons who treat patients with a cleft lip and cleft palate frequently perform nasal reconstructions at this age. *However, for most teens with nasal cosmetic issues, surgeons traditionally wait until roughly age 16.* The waiting is more about emotional stability than physical maturity. In certain emotionally charged situations, however, in which the nasal deformity is creating significant psychological havoc, a surgeon may consider earlier intervention. The teen and family must accept the possibility of revisional surgery if the nose continues to grow.

The next obstacle is to time the surgery so the teen has plenty of time to recover afterward. As noted earlier in the book, some activities will have to be postponed for a week or two, and others, like sports and exercise, for longer. Choose long vacations or transitional periods (such as the time between high school and college) for surgeries, especially if your teen is shy about sharing the experience with classmates. There is nothing like black and blue "shiners" to start the rumors flying about how your teenage son or daughter spent his or her vacation! Do not plan the surgery right before "Sweet 16" photos!

The Initial Consultation

At the initial consultation, a plastic surgeon should get to know the teen. By watching the way they move and speak, their body language can reveal much about how they view themselves. Are they shy? How do they relate to the family with them? Who is doing the talking? Who is dictating the problem and the solution? Is there something specific about their nose that is troublesome, or is there a more significant issue that is being attributed to the nose? As explained in previous chapters, for some, surgery resolves all related emotional troubles, but for others, in whom the problem lies deeper, surgery resolves nothing. A plastic surgeon experienced in the care of teens and adolescents can help both parent and teen evaluate the issues objectively and can make proper recommendations.

Once the ice is broken, the surgeon will ask what the teen would like "done" to the nose. Sometimes teens will bring in pictures of what they want. In the past, this was considered a red flag, foreshadowing unrealistic expectations. Today, many plastic surgeons see the pictures as a jumping-off point to begin a discussion and gain a frame of reference about the reality of their desires.

Some surgeons take photographs or send patients out for photographs and have them return later to look at the photos and draw out a plan. This practice has become old school with the advent of computer imaging. I prefer to immediately move to imaging and reviewing a treatment plan at the initial consultation. I need to know if the teen and the family and I are all on the same page. During this review of real-time images, I can show the patient and family what is possible and what I recommend and also demonstrate why doing more or less would be a bad idea. On the computer screen, bumps can be shaved, tips can be refined and rotated, and bridges can be narrowed, and we can see the "before" and "after" side by side.

Sometimes, the nose is the only part of the face that is out of proportion, and we can make a plan to refine it. Other times, the analysis of the nose as it relates to the face may reveal other imbalances in facial harmony such a small, recessive chin or shallow cheeks. The surgeon should point out these other issues and discuss them with the patient and family. Mutual understandings lead to the decisions most favorable and comfortable to the teen and family.

Once everyone agrees on a cosmetic plan, the nasal surgeon should fully evaluate the internal structures of the nose and the dental relationships of the face as well as the chin and the cheeks. A deviated nasal septum may present both an aesthetic structural and a functional problem and will need to be addressed. There may also be hypertrophy of the turbinates (swelling of the tissues that warm and humidify air passing through the nose). If the patient has a history of allergies, the surgeon should be aware of it, as this can affect an expected functional outcome. Surgery can realign nasal passages and remove blockages, but it does not cure allergies that can also cause nasal stuffiness and difficulty in breathing. Some patients also have dental issues that affect the appearance of the face. Orthodontic and even orthognathic (oral surgery) evaluations may be needed.

The initial consultation is also the appropriate time for the teen and family to make sure they're confident in their choice of surgeon. You should ask the surgeon the following questions (if he or she hasn't already answered them):

- Do you use computer imaging? Can you show me what to expect?
- May I see before-and-after photos of some of your patients?
- What technique will you use? Why?
- Where will the surgery be performed? Why?
- What type of anesthesia will be administered and by whom?
- Will there be packing? If so, when will it be removed?
- Are there functional aspects of the surgery that may be covered by insurance? What documentation do I need?
- Is it only my teen's nose that is the problem? Or is something else contributing to facial imbalance?

I touch on some of these points in more detail in the next sections.

Types of Nasal Surgery

In essence, the nose is a constellation of bone and cartilage. There is the bony pyramid at the bridge, which descends into a cartilage vault supported by a cartilage wingspan (the tip). Inside, there is a septal partition dividing the two air passages. On each side of the airway are the turbinates. Nasal surgery modifies some or all of these structures in some fashion.

Some surgeons use only an endonasal (internal incision) technique, and others use only an open (external nasal-base incision) technique. (See figure 7.2.) Many surgeons (including me) customize the approach based on the degree of deformity and the complexity of the reconstruction.

The original rhinoplasty—the one you or even your parents or siblings may have experienced twenty to forty years ago—was an internal, or closed, one. The reason it was considered such a difficult procedure to master was because the surgeon had to translate what he felt inside the nose to what he saw on the outside. In contrast, the external, or

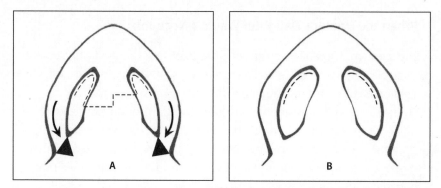

Figure 8.2 Placement of external incisions for open rhinoplasty (A) and internal incisions for closed rhinoplasty (B). The black triangles show a pattern to reduce nostril width.

open, approach allows the surgeon to see the nasal structures but adds a potentially visible scar. Both techniques have a place in rhinoplasty.

Simple bump reduction, tip thinning, and bridge narrowing are easily accomplished with the closed approach, particularly when all the structures are strong and well supported. When more detailed maneuvers are required to refine the nose and to strengthen weak or poorly supported tissues, the open approach is extremely valuable. Be aware that some surgeons have experience with only one type of approach. *Make sure your surgeon is adept at both methods so that he or she can take the best approach to your teen's particular problem.* Ask to see many before-and-after photos showing your teen's type of problem and its solution. Don't move forward until you are confident in your surgeon's abilities.

The Procedure and Recovery Time: What to Expect

For many teens this is their first surgery. Certain anxieties about the anesthesia and the venue for surgery are normal. Old-school nose jobs were performed under heavy sedation and local anesthesia. Today, many surgeons want the patient asleep and the airway protected from any bleeding. I agree with this and put all my nasal surgery patients under general anesthesia. It takes the patient "out of the loop," quells anxiety, and allows the surgeon to work undisturbed.

Nasal surgeries usually take between two and three hours, but find out your surgeon's timetable so you do not worry needlessly as the minutes pass. Fewer and fewer surgeons place gauze packing into the nose after the

When the Doctor's Daughter Wants a Nose Job

The questions I posed for you earlier in the book to ask yourself when considering plastic surgery for your teen are the very same ones I asked myself when confronted by two of my daughters' desire for rhinoplasty.

They were several years apart in age, and each made an independent decision to request surgery. There were no breathing problems to camouflage their wants for cosmetic improvement. They both had inherited the family trait of a large nose on a small face. Each felt it was dominating their face, and that made them unhappy with their looks.

This was an interesting and complicated problem for me because I was both an objective surgeon looking at what could be done (and what I have done for decades for others) and a subjective parent believing that my children were beautiful as they were. And, like any parent, I had a desire to protect them from anything "unnecessary."

My children were familiar with my work and wanted me to be their doctor; they would not accept another. From my perspective, if I was the chosen surgeon by many people they have known over the years how could I not be part of their care?

Computer imaging was the most beneficial tool in our discussion and decision-making process. It showed them how I viewed their noses and the improvements I could realistically make without sacrificing their individuality and identity—basically, it illustrated what I was willing to do. I answered each of their questions carefully and concluded that I could realistically and safely perform the surgeries with time for them to recover without disrupting their academic and athletic schedules.

It was only after mutual agreement between each teen and her mother and me that we took next step. I have a certified operating facility and a very skilled staff of nurses and anesthesiologists. I knew my kids would be in the safest of hands, and that would allow me to do my job.

As I drove my children to the operating suite, I felt two things: anxiety over whether or not they would be happy with their new look, and satisfaction that as both a surgeon and a parent I had done my due diligence in preparing everyone for the event.

The results were as I'd planned, and their responses were gratifying.

Experiencing in my own household the aftermath of the procedures helped me as a doctor, because seeing the recovery firsthand—twice—gave

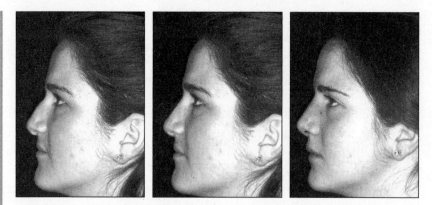

My 16-year-old girl with a nasal deformity before and after surgery. The middle picture depicts the computer mock up. The final result, as shown on the right, closely resembles the proposed plan.

me a fresh perspective on patient healing. My daughters' discomfort with the nasal packing convinced me to abandon a long-applied tradition and eliminate it from future surgeries. Watching their responses as the splints were removed and the swelling subsided gave me insight into helping patients through the transition period. I photo-documented each week of the recovery. This became a very valuable tool in showing other patients what to expect. Additionally, future patients and their parents found it reassuring that I trusted myself and my staff enough to treat to my own children.

surgery, although some still do. Ask about this, and, if your surgeon does it, ask when the packing will be removed. Rhinoplasty patients usually wear a nasal splint (a cast on the nose) for a week. During that time, patients should be at home resting with their head elevated to decrease swelling.

When your surgeon removes the splint, you should expect swelling and bruising, even though the extent of it varies from patient to patient. Teens can now usually resume their social and academic schedules, but sports and other strenuous activities are prohibited for another month, when the nose will be solidly healed. Remember, it takes months for the complete resolution of swelling and for the nose to assume the final shape achieved on the operating table and the one that will last a lifetime.

Secondary Surgeries

In spite of best efforts, about 10 percent of rhinoplasties need revision, according to national statistics. For most, the revisional surgery is a simple touch-up with little risk or downtime. And indeed it is better to have undercorrected a nose than to have overcorrected it. Most surgeons will not charge an additional fee for the second surgery and consider it part of the overall job. But in some situations, it can be more complicated, especially if a new surgeon becomes involved.

Many experienced nasal surgeons have been called for a second opinion when a patient's surgery has yielded poor results. Most of these were overdone surgeries where the original surgeon was married to a singular technique that did not match up with the uniqueness of the patient. This causes a great deal of anxiety for the teen and parents, as well as for the surgeon now asked to fix the problem. Many surgeons will not take on another's troubles for fear of inheriting the anger that goes with the frustration and the additional expense. Personally, I take a deep breath and remind myself that I should use my skill and compassion to help restore self-esteem, and therefore I do take on revision cases like this.

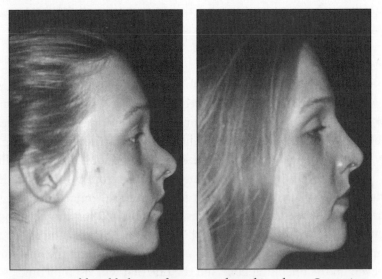

Restoration of facial balance after an overdone rhinoplasty. Correction was with a bone graft to normalize nasal height.

Families need to know that major revisional nasal surgery is challenging. It often involves adding back bone and cartilage that has been injudiciously removed. This means robbing Peter to pay Paul. The needed tissues must be taken from like sources: cartilage from the septum, ears, or ribs; and bone from the hip, ribs, or skull. Foreign materials like silicone should be avoided. They do not fare well in the nose and can potentially lead to infections at unpredictable times. Most revisional surgeries utilize the external, or open, approach. This allows the surgeon to see what has happened and to deconstruct the problem to provide a correct reconstruction.

I treated a young college freshman who had undergone six nasal surgeries between ages 16 and 18; each surgery had left her worse than the one before. Finally, the original surgeon had given up. Needless to say, her frustration level was high and her finances low. I agreed to reconstruct her nose. It was a complicated process to remove the irregular cartilages as well as the accumulated scar tissue and to rebuild the height and tip of the nose. She was so emotionally worn down, as were her parents, that in spite of a very successful outcome, it was hard for them to really appreciate it.

I do not describe this scenario to frighten teens away from the procedure. I included it to stress that nose jobs, as common as they are, need to be approached seriously, and you should have the utmost confidence in the surgeon you choose before proceeding.

Insurance Coverage

Gone are those days when the mere term "deviated septum" equated with insurance payment for a nose job. Now it is very hard to obtain coverage, and many legitimate cases are denied. Certainly, cosmetic situations will not ever be covered. For those with breathing problems, insurance companies often ask for six months of conservative treatments like allergy evaluations and humidifiers as well as the use of nasal sprays (even though repeated use of these sprays is in fact harmful to the membranes of the nose) before they will consider covering a surgery. Some companies require second opinions and CAT scans to document structural problems. If your teen has a breathing problem, be prepared to obtain documentation from allergists, otolaryngologists, and radiologists. Do not try to fake a functional problem to obtain coverage.

It usually does not succeed, and surgery under the guise of improving breathing when your nose functions are normal could be harmful. Even if you obtain coverage for a functional problem, it is generally only a partial reimbursement. The insurance company will expect you to pay for aspects it deems cosmetic, including the hospital fees and the anesthesiologist.

Evaluating the Face

In many ways, the chin and cheeks complete the face and define its personality. In the very young face, the chin is small and the cheeks full. As the face grows, so does the chin, revealing a strong facial profile. With age, many chins sag and the cheeks diminish in size as volume is lost.

The chin and cheeks are an essential part of the analysis of facial balance. This may come as a surprise to many teens and parents who are focused on a nose job as the primary facial plastic surgical issue. It is important for you and your teen to have an open mind when the plastic surgeon evaluates your teen's face. Do not take the analysis as a criticism but rather as a proposal that could give your teen the best possible results. You would not want your surgeon to withhold his true thoughts on what your child needs, and your surgeon doesn't want to correct a nose only to end up with a patient who is still unhappy with his face. Thus, it's best for the surgeon to bring up his recommendations

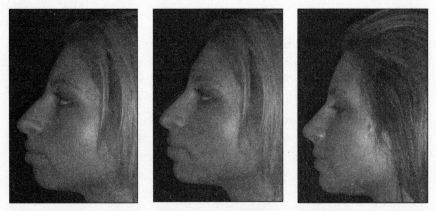

Facial imbalance consisting of large nose, small chin, and flat cheeks. Center photo is the computer work plan. The third is the final result, closely resembling the imaged ideal.

for discussion to help you make the most informed decision. Although some surgeons are guilty of trying to create their own "my fair lady" (known as the "Pygmalion effect") by achieving what they want in spite of patient desires, most moral and ethical surgeons want to hear what patients want and then advise accordingly.

Plastic surgeons who are adept at facial structural surgery can rapidly assess what a face may need to be balanced and proportionate. Sometimes the solution requires a team approach including orthodonture and even maxillofacial surgery when the jaw needs major structural change. Other times simple augmentations can provide balance. It could be that work on the chin alone will give the face harmony. Or perhaps just the cheeks need refinement. A good plastic surgeon seeks to do the least and to provide the most.

Chin Surgery

If your teen's jaw is significantly out of proportion to the rest of his or her face, and there are problems with dental bite, significant jaw surgery (orthognathic surgery) may be required. This is usually performed by an oral–maxillofacial surgeon and will precede any plan for nasal refinements.

Most often balance issues center around a small or recessive chin (see figure 8.3). Because many teens have already had braces, they are not looking for extensive surgery on their lower jaw, and their parents, who have spent a small fortune on those braces, certainly are not either. If the teeth and dental occlusion are in place, then the surgeon will likely suggest other procedures to advance the profile. These could include cutting and moving forward the bony chin point, inserting chin implants, or adding fillers such as fat grafts.

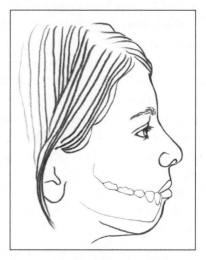

Figure 8.3 The chin is retruded, throwing off the balance of the face.

Sliding Genioplasty

Cutting and advancing the bone is called a sliding genioplasty. Surgical techniques for this are sophisticated, and results are very predictable and can be planned in advance with computer programming. The surgeon makes the incision inside the mouth at the base of the lip and gum line, giving access to the bone. Once the bone is cut it is advanced forward and positioned as planned and then secured with very small plates and screws. (See figure 8.4.)

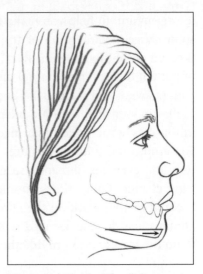

Figure 8.4 Results of a sliding genioplasty, in which the bone is cut and advanced.

Chin Implants

In my experience, unless the chin is significantly receded, most teens are not looking for involved surgery and will reject an additional procedure if they perceive it as a major intervention. In these cases, I suggest a chin implant for augmentation.

Implants come in a range of sizes and shapes and can be contoured to the face. Surgery to insert an implant is called onlay surgery, as the implant is placed on top of the existing bone to increase its projection. Incisions for chin implants can be either inside the mouth (as for a sliding genioplasty) or on the outside beneath the chin. Your surgeon will have a preference about the incision, and you should discuss this in advance. (If, however, your teen is having a small liposuction in conjunction with an

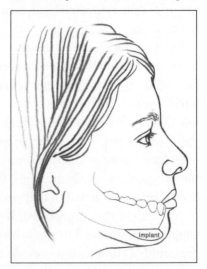

Figure 8.5 A chin implant (most often silicone) used as an "onlay" advancement.

implant to further define the neck and chin, the incision will be external under the chin.)

Chin implant surgery is a common and straightforward procedure, but afterward, the patient can experience bruising and swelling and some temporary numbness of the lower lip. When the incision is inside the mouth, eating and teeth brushing are limited immediately after surgery. But these effects go away within days, and patients feel better. (See figure 8.5.)

Fat Grafting

Sometimes even the suggestion of a chin implant raises eyebrows with parents. Although silicone implants have withstood the test of time, they still may be rejected as too invasive or complicated. In these situations, I encourage the technique of fat grafting. The fat is taken from the teen's own body, and the recovery is virtually painless.

Fat has the unique ability to mimic the tissues it is placed against. When used in chin augmentations and placed along the jawline, it feels like bone. According to national statistics, more than 50 percent of the fat remains five years after surgery. Although this may seem like a negative, it can be a benefit for the patient because it allows him to "try out" the advancement. If he likes it, more fat can be added if needed, and if he doesn't (which is rare), the fat will slowly reabsorb.

The procedure is simple and involves borrowing a small quantity of fat from wherever it is available—usually the hips or abdomen. (And, no, it is not enough for a "free liposuction"—it is such a small amount you will never know it is missing!) The fat is processed to remove the water and oil components and then injected into the chin area with small needles. Patients never complain of pain and are pleased

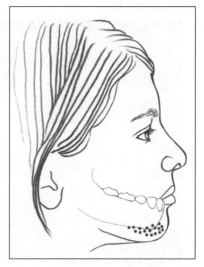

Figure 8.6 Fat is transferred into the chin in front of the bone to build out the projection.

that they made the choice to do it, especially when they see their before and after photos. (See figure 8.6.)

The Cheeks

Many teens do not realize that the phenomenon of "flat cheeks" can have a plastic surgical solution. All they know is that they feel like they look tired. This is because a flattened mid-facial region is a sign of aging. When it occurs in teens, it is a facial imbalance issue that can be corrected with long-term results. The addition of volume in this area can brighten the face and improve the proportion to the nose and chin.

Once again, the choices for augmentation can include implants or fillers. I prefer to use fat as the filler because it is simple to inject and is readily available, especially when already harvested for the chin. An interim or temporary solution for those still unsure about changing their chin and cheeks is to use a filler substance like Radiesse (hydroxyapatite), Restylane (hyaluronic acid), or Juvéderm (hyaluronic acid). These "volumizers" will provide the desired effect but will last only months. If the teen and parent now see the value of the surgeon's suggestions for facial balance, they can consider one of the other procedures—fat grafting or implants.

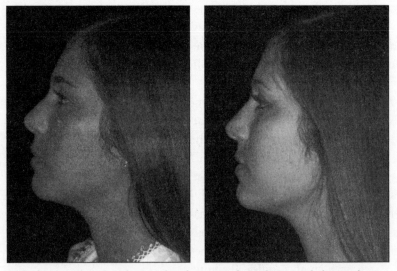

Facial balancing procedure with refinement rhinoplasty, and chin and cheek augmentation with fat grafting. Multiple small changes can make a big difference.

Final Thoughts

Facial imbalances that occur through puberty as the teen develops a mature face can cause a significant amount of emotional distress. It is best not to run away from discussion of the problem but to seek professional advice on behalf of your teen. Once you and your teen have explored the various options, you can make a knowledgeable decision.

It is important to empower your teen but not push or enable them. They must want the procedure(s) for themselves. It is not enough to offer plastic surgery because you the parent may have had it. If a parent has had plastic surgery, this does not mean the child necessarily needs plastic surgery. I have seen more than one teen brought in by their parents because the child's nose was significantly different from their noses. What the teen was unaware of was that both parents had rhinoplasties in their youth. These children did not have a frame of reference for their own familial traits. They just knew they were different. And the parents wanted correction to protect their own vanities and to keep their own surgeries secret.

It is also important for teens to understand that structural surgeries like these require time for healing and for swelling to settle. What you see initially is not what you get. Teens must accept the time frame for recovery and comply with the surgeon's instructions to see the results the surgeon intended.

Parents need to be prepared for the unexpected after surgery. A teen's reaction to the results may be unpredictable. I have seen elation, surprise, anxiety, and even shock as the teens adjusted to their new look. It is important to realize that for most of us, the face that is reflected in the mirror is "us." When it changes, a psychological adjustment is often necessary. Some teens even go through a period of sadness and regret as their physical wounds heal. The entire team—surgeon and family—should provide support. Occasionally, a teen may need psychological intervention to help get through this transition period.

What I have seen, more often than not, is a life-changing and positive result that reinforces a teen's self-esteem and sets the stage for adulthood founded on a healthy self-image.

9

Breasts and Chests: A Delicate Balance

☞ Breast reduction has the highest satisfaction rate of any plastic surgery.

☞ Breast implants for teens are not approved by the FDA except under very unique circumstances like extreme underdevelopment. A decision to have this surgery should never be taken lightly.

☞ Breast surgery with or without implants has never been the cause of cancer.

☞ Inverted nipples and nipple damage form piercings are common and can be fixed with minimally invasive surgery.

Megan and her friends are shopping for prom dresses. The girls are excitedly grabbing gowns from the racks, holding them in front of themselves, and imagining the reaction that the form-fitting, strapless sheaths of silk will provoke.

"Come on, Megan, what do you want to try on?"

Megan looks down, suddenly quiet. "Oh, I don't know," she mutters, pulling her jacket close around her and feeling suddenly very vulnerable. "I'll find something."

Her friends trot off to the dressing room, chattering happily while Megan looks at the racks. Nothing for her here. All these gowns are strapless, and there's no way Megan is going to fit into one of these with her double-D bust.

She feels embarrassed, angry, and helpless. Her friends are calling for her to join them. Megan grabs a matronly black dress two sizes too big and heads for the fitting room. Once inside, she makes sure she finds a stall to herself while the other girls dress together in one of the larger rooms. She tries on the dress. It's way too large, but at least it slims down her bust. Megan feels decades older than her 16 years.

That night she goes home, sits in front of the TV, and eats a pint of ice cream. Her mom notices there's something wrong but can't figure out what it is. She's a perfectly normal, lovely teenage girl—but with a problem that affects millions of women around the world: macromastia, or overly developed, heavy breasts. Her figure has defined her as "different" since she was 13.

This story is a composite example of situations teens tell me about on a regular basis. Fortunately, the problem has a surgical solution.

PERHAPS NO BODY PART defines feminine desires for plastic surgery more than breasts. Indeed, much of the controversy in the media stems from the myriad tales of young girls getting their breasts augmented through implants—a practice that is not only fraught with problems but is also against the FDA's strict guidelines about cosmetic breast surgery for minors. (There are some cases in which implants for teens are reasonable and approved, and we'll go into them later.)

For the most part, the surgeries that make sense for teenagers are those that address overly large breasts on girls (macromastia) and on boys (gynecomastia), breast asymmetry, and nipple problems. Let me assure you at the outset that, no matter what you may have heard to the contrary, breast cancer has never been attributed to breast surgery with or without implants. The FDA has also concluded that there are no immunologic risks to the presence of silicone implants. So although breast reduction for teens (and in some rare cases, breast augmentation) is invasive and not to be considered lightly, it does not increase your teen's chances of getting breast cancer.

Macromastia: When Bigger Is Not Better

The surgery that has the highest satisfaction rate of any major plastic surgical procedure is breast reduction for macromastia. You may have seen stories in *People* magazine and in other media outlets about celebrity breast reductions like those done on Drew Barrymore and Queen Latifah. Though these celebs were adults when they had the surgery, they give a good idea of the before-and-after looks.

Drew Barrymore is a small-framed woman with breasts that were too large for her size. The plastic surgeon reduced them to a size more in keeping with her petite frame, probably about a B cup. But macromastia doesn't affect just small-framed people. Queen Latifah is queen-sized—a large-framed woman with broad shoulders—but her breasts far outweighed the rest of her body. Her breasts were reduced in proportion to her size from a triple D to a C-D. The comparison illustrates that the goal is not to give a girl one particular acceptable size but to give her a size that is fitting for her body frame and structure.

How to Know If There's a Problem

There are not always obvious visual cues to the problem. Some girls, when they develop overly heavy breasts, will hide them in baggy clothes and sometimes even become overweight or crash diet as a reaction to the "fat" part of them they can't control. Parents should be on the lookout for these behaviors. In some families, big breasts might be a family trait or something considered to be a plus, but the teen may in fact be deeply unhappy with them. Parents should consider their teen's feelings on the matter.

Other clues to a problem include physical issues: Your teen may be suffering back or neck pain. Even shooting pains down the arm and numbness from nerve compressions can occur as a result of the heavy stress that overly large breasts place on the body. If your teen is having problems participating in gym class or is limited in sports, and you suspect her breasts might be an issue, they probably are. It's not easy doing jumping jacks when your breasts are doing most of the bouncing!

Occasionally, the problem is solely a result of being overweight and will clear up when the teen loses weight. But a teen who is heavily proportioned on top and thinner elsewhere may not be able to lose enough weight to correct the condition. Asking a teen to diet constantly when the issue is not overall weight but weight distribution is a losing battle. The constant dieting can also be unhealthy because it can lead to issues like anorexia and body dysmorphic disorder. A teen will see images of a celebrity like Nicole Richie, who lost her full bust when she lost a lot of weight, and want to do the same thing. Dieting down to an unhealthy weight is not the solution to macromastia.

The Surgical Solution to Macromastia: Breast-Reduction Surgery

Breast-reduction surgery is straightforward and time-tested. It is designed to decrease the volume and improve the shape of the breasts. There are many techniques, each having its own proponents, but they all basically shift the position of the nipple/areola complex into a visually pleasing position and then reduce the breast tissue around it. (We discuss the different techniques in more detail below.) The effect is smaller and younger-looking breasts more fitting to a teen. Young women who have had to shop in misses departments can suddenly be juniors again. Ugly, heavy-strapped bras can be tossed for thin-strapped, "cute" ones. As one of my patients, 18-year-old Valerie, noted:

> "Going into Victoria's Secret and buying a bra off the rack was a mere dream until my breast reduction surgery. I wanted to feel like other teenage girls but also to be comfortable in my own skin, but the strain of my large breasts, physical and emotional, made that impossible. I've never regretted the surgery and feel lucky that I had the support of my family."

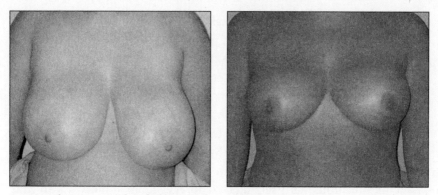

Breast reduction providing balance and proportion.

The Consultation

From the initial phone call to the office, the staff should be concerned with the emotional, physical, and financial well-being of the prospective patient and family. The teen has most likely been inundated with ideas on plastic surgery from Internet and other media sources, and there will likely be plenty of information to confirm or dispel.

When the teen comes to my office, I first have a general discussion with her to learn about her life and to determine why and how her breast size is interfering with it. I want to know when breast growth began and if it has been stable. I also want to ascertain if there are any growth and development conditions that need evaluation prior to surgery as well as any other medical conditions that might preclude or defer consideration of surgery.

Next, there is the sensitive and embarrassing obstacle of the physical exam to overcome. Often girls with overly large breasts are embarrassed by them, making the exam emotionally trying. The surgeon should be very clear and compassionate about the exam procedure. A nurse must always be in the room, and if the teen wishes it, her mother can be present as well.

Once I have examined the patient's breasts, I can begin to outline a work plan. In my initial evaluation with the teen and her parent, I will sometimes illustrate the technique I plan to use by drawing a temporary, washable outline of the proposed incision pattern on the patient. This allows the teen and parent to envision the operative plan and to

135

be reminded that there will be incisions and therefore scars. I transfer this outline to a model in a booklet put out by the American Society of Plastic Surgeons for them to take home as a reference.

Before the consultation is over, I review in detail what the surgery entails, including the risks and recovery time involved. All breast surgeries carry some risk, including infection, bleeding, alteration in nipple sensation, possible inability to breast-feed, even an unfavorable aesthetic result. Although the risks are very low, they need to be openly discussed; you'll want to be sure to talk to your surgeon about the potentially necessary rectifications with secondary and revisional surgery. I also find it imperative to let my patient and her family know about how much time the procedure and recovery will take. Some surgeons deliberately underestimate surgical and healing time so as not to alarm a patient. I believe this does more harm than being honest. If the family knows the surgeon's track record for time, they will accept it. If they are expecting the surgery to be over sooner than is realistic, they will be worried when the procedure takes longer.

Your surgeon should discuss the issues of insurance reimbursement for the procedure. The size of the breasts in relation to the overall size of the patient often determines if an insurance company will consider the problem functional enough for coverage, along with cup size, back pain, and skin irritations. Documentation of these and photographic proof is very important and needs to be sent to insurance providers.

Techniques

The size of the breasts determines what incision pattern will be the most ideal. These can range from the vertical-pattern, or "lollipop," incision (which I use most often) to the more traditional anchor, or inverted-T, incision (reserved for larger and lower breasts) to the occasional "free nipple graft" technique, in which the nipples are detached from the breasts and then repositioned and reattached. (See figure 9.1.) This last technique is needed only in rare cases in which the breasts are so large and low that nipple viability could be compromised if pedicle techniques (those in which the nipple is not removed) were used.

Your physician will evaluate your daughter's case to determine which method is best, but usually for teens, the free nipple graft is not used and the less-invasive "lollipop" incision is preferred.

Figure 9.1 These illustrations show the types of breast reduction incisions and techniques. From top to bottom: the anchor, or inverted-T, pattern with a pedicle ("tongue") of breast tissue to preserve nipple sensation and circulation; the vertical, or "lollipop," pattern with a pedicle to maintain viability of the nipple; the "free nipple graft" technique for reduction of very large breasts when a pedicle may not be successful in preserving viability of the nipple.

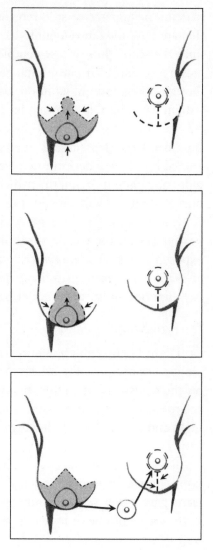

Risks and Trade-offs

Breast-reduction surgery, like all body-contouring surgery, has risks and trade-offs that the teen and her family need to understand.

As with any surgery, there is a risk of bleeding. The need for a blood transfusion for a patient undergoing a breast reduction is rare but not unheard of. To eliminate the possible risk of blood-borne disease, patients can bank their own blood in advance of the surgery so that it is available in case of emergency. There is also a risk of delayed bleeding after the surgery, and the need to return to the operating room.

Breast-reduction surgery requires incisions, and that means scars. Plastic surgeons today are better than ever at minimizing them, but it is not a scarless surgery. And scars are not always predictable. The most common scars are the "lollipop" scars that go around the areola to the bottom of the front of the breast. "Anchor" scars, which add scars to the bottom of the breast (where the underwire is in a bra), used to be more common but are still frequently used. Incision patterns should be discussed in advance Surgeons may give patients postoperative scar remedies, like crèmes and silicone sheets, that are easy and convenient to use. However, these products only minimize the scars; they cannot completely remove them.

Surgery can also cause changes in nipple sensation and erection, though this is rare. In addition, there is always the possibility that the patient won't be able to breast-feed. I always tell families that if they are dedicated members of La Leche League, then they might not be good candidates for this surgery. Surgeons can't predict how the surgically altered nipple will perform in a breast-feeding situation. I tell all breast-reduction patients that if the pedicled (attached) nipple is compromised during surgery, I will convert it to a free nipple graft.

All in all, however, breast reduction remains one of the most popular procedures on the plastic surgeon's menu. To a girl who is constantly exposed to sexual scrutiny because of her overly large breasts, the risks of surgery are worth it to finally feel like a teen again—to have people pay attention to *her* and not her breasts.

The Procedure

I perform breast-reduction surgeries in the hospital with an anesthesiologist because it is the safest approach for all concerned. Depending on their postsurgical status, many teens can go home from the recovery room the same day as the surgery, but some will elect to stay the night and go home the following day. I always leave this decision to the family.

All the removed breast tissue must be sent for pathological evaluation. This serves as a reassurance that the breasts are healthy, since most teens have never had a mammogram. (Once, a cancer was discovered in the tissue of one of my patients, so the procedure was life-saving as well.)

Recovery

The patient must work as a team with her surgeon, and that means following instruction for recovery. She must rest. Often the recovery is remarkably painless. Teens feel good fast—within hours—and want to get out and about faster than their body may be prepared for. When I discuss the procedure with teens and families during the initial consultation, the topic of recovery is always the most difficult part of the discussion. Some surgeons will minimize recovery to close the deal. I am open and honest because I believe that if the patient and family know what to expect, it minimizes problems in the long term.

During surgery, I use absorbable sutures, so there is nothing to remove later. I rarely use drains but many surgeons use them out of habit. (They must be kept clean and checked at specific intervals until they can be removed, usually a day or so after surgery). My dressing is a support bra that holds the breasts over small tapes on the incisions. I see the patient two times a week for the first three weeks to change the bandages myself. The patient is allowed to bathe up to the bra or take brief "back"showers as soon after surgery as she'd like.

By three weeks after the surgery, patients are ready to resume normal daily activities except for gym and sports. I prescribe six weeks of abstaining from sports. I keep track of the teen for at least one year to observe the fading of the scars and the shape of the breasts. Teens will be aging, and so will their breasts. They need to be informed that with time the shape may change, and so may the size once pregnancy and weight changes occur. Another possible postsurgical development is "bottoming out," in which the breast gets fuller at the base. Usually, this is of a minor aesthetic concern; occasionally, a small revision is needed. If the teen is happy with the result, nothing need be done.

Breast reductions usually result in a very positive quality-of-life change. Suddenly, a teen feels and looks like her peers, not a woman twenty years older. Sexual innuendos cease, and physical activity becomes easier. For a girl with clinically overdeveloped breasts, there is very little downside to this procedure. I feel a great deal of pride and happiness when I review the hundreds of successful breast reductions I have done through the years for teenage girls. Their lives have invariably benefited in many ways: physically, psychologically, and socially. Armed with the information provided here, parents can give their teen the gift of a lifetime: freedom from back, arm, shoulder, and neck pain and a body that does not limit her socially or physically.

Gynecomastia: Why Jimmy Won't Take His Shirt Off

Girls are supposed to have breasts. Boys are supposed to have chests. Sometimes nature interferes and boys develop breasts. The condition of male breasts is called gynecomastia, and it is often the cause of cruel teasing and deep emotional distress for boys.

If you suspect that your teen is having this issue, look at his lifestyle. Does he shirk from sports in which boys have to strip off their shirts? Does he cut gym class often? Does he tend to wear loose and dark clothing? Although it is an embarrassing and emotionally charged subject, it is important to talk to your teen to determine if this issue is at the heart of some of his behavior. Shame is not an option here. This is a condition that may have medical causes and one that has an easy surgical solution when other factors are ruled out.

June, the mother of one of my patients, puts the situation in perspective:

"My son, around the age of 13, developed a breast on one side. He became very self-conscious. I discovered it when he refused to go with the family on warm-weather vacations. When I realized there was a surgical solution to the problem, I presented it to my son, who felt like a weight of shame was lifted from him. He had the surgery and soon went back to being a 'normal' teen. Now the whole family goes on vacation together!"

The reason for gynecomastia is often an imbalance of hormones. Certain medications (including anabolic steroids used for bodybuilding) and even marijuana can be the culprits. The problem can also be mimicked by pubescent weight gain or obesity. A thorough medical evaluation is necessary. Once the problem is defined and the causes known, a solution can follow, whether it is an alteration in medications, a change in diet and exercise, a no-pot policy, or surgery. It is important to get to the root of the problem to prevent future overgrowth. When gynecomastia has been diagnosed and nonsurgical options eliminated, surgery is often the best and most realistic solution to the problem.

The Surgical Solution to Gynecomastia

As with other plastic surgery, the initial consultation requires a physical exam. Boys are typically embarrassed about this, especially when their mothers are present. They most often do not want to be viewed by other females, including nurses, so I usually have my female nurse stand outside the door until invited in. You may want to discuss this issue with your plastic surgeon before you take your child in for his exam.

The initial consultation with your plastic surgeon will help define the type of correction that will work best for your teen. In some cases, when the "breast" is fatty, liposculpture may be all that is required. In others, when the tissue is glandular and fibrous, direct removal through a tiny incision around the nipple may be needed. A combination of procedures is also possible.

The surgery is done as an outpatient procedure under general anesthesia or local anesthesia with sedation. I usually perform the surgery

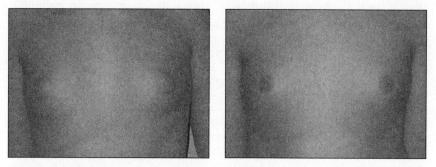

Fatty gynecomastia corrected with liposuction through small "poke hole" incisions in the sides of the breasts.

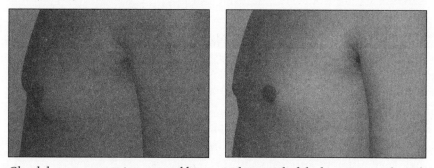

Glandular gynecomastia corrected by surgical removal of the breast tissue through a small inconspicuous incision around the lower nipple area.

Developing Chest Muscles Sans Surgery

I also want to stress that the purpose of surgery for gynecomastia is to normalize the appearance of a male's chest, not to implant anything or accentuate the "pecs." Chest implants for teen boys is not only dangerous, it's against good practice as defined by the FDA.

Once a boy has normalized his chest to a typically male appearance, workouts and sports can help give a more defined look—but it should be natural, not enhanced by implants or steroids.

in my own surgical center, primarily because I have sophisticated liposuction equipment not often found in hospitals. The procedure differs from female breast reduction because it can involve purely liposuction, purely glandular removal, or both. Incisions are minimal in size, and no drains are needed. Recovery is quick and relatively painless. The dressing is a compression vest. Boys are back in school in days and can switch from the vest to commercially available compression garments (such as those made by Under Armour) that look like normal clothing for privacy while healing. This is a plus since the compression is needed for about six weeks.

Once healed, the teenage boy's chest will be just like those of other boys—the problem virtually vanishes, and a lifetime of shame and emotional and physical withdrawal has been averted. When the patient's chest has normalized, he may use workouts and sports to give it a more defined look (however, he should do it naturally, not with implants or steroids). As with female breast reduction, there is a high degree of satisfaction with this type of surgery.

Asymmetry: Putting Nature Back in Balance

Most people think breasts are supposed to be twins—and identical twins at that. Although most women's breasts are not perfectly symmetrical, there are some cases in which one breast develops differently and produces an extremely asymmetrical appearance. In fact, it's more common than you'd imagine. Asymmetrical breasts come in many variations, and they have different surgical solutions.

When one breast is larger than the other, but the smaller breast is of adequate size, then a simple reduction–matching procedure is in order. This is the easiest of problems to resolve. It does not involve breast implants.

Other times, the problem is more complex: one breast may be way too large and the other way too small. A reduction alone is not enough. The smaller breast requires an augmentation. This is one of the only situations in which augmentation is green-lighted by the FDA for those younger than 18. Purely cosmetic augmentations are not approved for minors, but the correction of asymmetrical breasts does meet the standards for implant use. Parents and teens, however, need to know that the surgery involves implanting a foreign object—an FDA-approved breast implant—into the body. Patients must be diligent about having yearly exams, and the family needs to know that supplementary surgery to correct changes from breast growth or shifting of the implant may be necessary as well as the possible "wearing out" of the implant.

The Surgical Solution to Asymmetrical Breasts

The most critical part of the solution to breast asymmetry is formulating a satisfying plan. This is easiest when one breast merely needs to be matched. When both breasts need work, sometimes the surgery can get complex, even if implants are not needed. Both breasts may need reduction but in different amounts. One may need to be lifted and the other reduced. Or one may require an implant for size and shape. Asymmetry, by its very nature, doesn't follow any set rules, and surgical solutions vary widely depending on the circumstances.

When approaching a teen with an asymmetry issue, I use a system devised by the ancient Greek scientist Archimedes, who used water displacement to determine weight. By "dipping" each breast into a large graduated cylinder filled with water, I can ascertain the weight of each breast and the difference between them. The measurements are accurate and useful in planning the surgery to balance the breasts, whether it be reduction or augmentation. The method also demonstrates to the teen and her family that I am not flying by the seat of my pants but have a plan with a scientific basis.

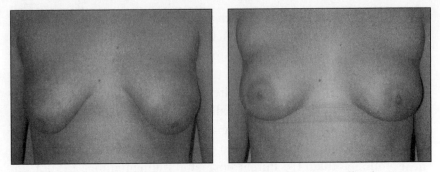

Breast asymmetry corrected with an uplift (mastopexy) and a small reduction.

As with other breast surgeries, I mark the patient for surgery in advance in my office, with my nurse. This allows for more questions to be answered and for the plan to be reviewed. If both breasts are undergoing surgery, the smaller breast is adjusted first. This sets the size for the reduction of the larger. If an implant is used only on one side, the adjusted breasts may look the same after surgery, but they are not. They will age differently and refinement may be needed over time. A reminder: This is a procedure that requires a lifetime of maintenance and the teen and parents need to be aware of that fact before committing to it.

It is the worst feeling in the world when you don't look like the other girls. I could not wear bathing suits, tank tops, or any strapless dresses. I had to put different size pads in my bras to balance my markedly different-sized breasts. I became depressed, gained weight, and was feeling sick on a regular basis.

As soon as I had a consultation and realized that there was hope for normalcy, my depression lessened. After the surgery, which for me was the summer before my freshman year of high school, I felt much more comfortable in my own body. I began to work out. I lost weight and went out for school sports.

—Marie, age 15

My daughter Marie had been severely emotionally affected by her breast deformity. It began at puberty and got progressively worse. We endured many difficult times in the summer months when bathing suits needed to be worn or whenever the locker room needed to be utilized. It was as if she'd had a mastectomy on one side. Self-esteem and body image are very important no matter our age.

    After the surgery, an augmentation on one side and a reduction on the other, Marie began to feel better physically and emotionally. Even her irritable bowel syndrome has improved. The mind and body are connected!

—Jane (mother)

Breast Lifts and Breast Augmentation for Special Cases

Sometimes even a young person is faced with sagging breasts, a condition called mammary ptosis. The condition is usually caused by age or maternity, but occasionally, a young person will be saddled with naturally slack breasts from first development. The issue, of course, creates emotional, psychological, and social interaction problems. Imagine dressing for gym and having all the other girls stare at your chest or not being able to wear the same types of bras your friends are wearing because you need the support that a 40-year-old woman requires.

A breast lift, or mastopexy, is the repositioning of the nipple/areola complex and repackaging of the breast tissue into a smaller envelope. The procedure is performed as an outpatient surgery, usually under general anesthesia. The benefits are significant, the outcome predictably positive, and the risks small. The biggest issue for a teen to deal with

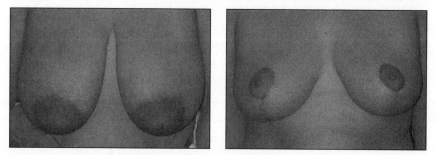

Teenager with significant sagging of breasts with mastopexy correction with areolar reduction.

is the trade-off of scars for shape—a trade-off that I have rarely seen declined.

> Thank you for helping me. I am a tenth grader who had breasts that look like an old lady. What teenager has droopy, saggy breasts? How was I supposed to act and feel young when the mirror was showing me different? How was I to deal with the fact that only surgery would balance my shape? I feel good about my body now and have nothing to hide.
> —Rory, age 16

In other cases, teens are faced with the fact that they have no breast development at all. Only in these most severe cases should breast implants be considered for young teens. The FDA disapproves of breast augmentation in most minors for good reason: Many girls are emotionally driven before they are physically developed. They have images of themselves and their breasts that time will temper. Therefore breast augmentation, for purely "cosmetic" reasons, is not permitted until age 18. (Of course, there are unscrupulous surgeons who will bend the rules, and the press is full of stories of these cases.)

If you have been reading this book from the beginning, you know that I believe my position as a plastic surgeon is to benefit my patient's health. I follow the principal rule we are all taught in medical school: "First, do no harm." This instruction to "never do harm" was even written in the Hippocratic Oath and passed down to every surgeon since that time, and I often wonder if some of my colleagues have forgotten it. I will not delve further into that issue except to warn families of teens to do their homework. Do not look for a plastic surgeon who will satisfy your teen's

"It is important to get the message out to the media that there is a distinction between breast augmentation for purely cosmetic enhancement and those in need for more serious conditions."

— Dr. Richard D'Amico, a past president of the American Society for Plastic Surgeons

146

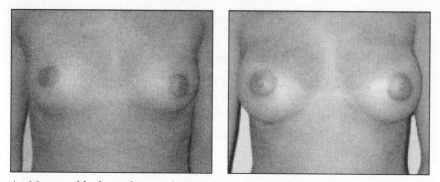

An 18-year-old who underwent breast augmentation between high school and college.

By the time I was 13 years old I was miserable! Where were my breasts? By 16 they were still barely an "A" cup and based on genetics were not [going to get] much bigger. I tried padded bras but was ridiculed for "stuffing." I begged for breast implants. I saw a program about a doctor who specialized in teenage self-esteem issues and I convinced my parents to at least allow a consultation. That was one of the best days of my life.

My doctor agreed that my breasts were disproportionately small. He was in favor of breast-augmentation surgery but with many stipulations. I had to continue to see my therapist. I had to quit smoking and start exercising. And he would only do it in the transition period between high school and college.

My renewed sense of hope allowed the time to pass, and I met all his criteria.

Two days after graduation I had the procedure. I went from barely an "A" to a full "B." It was a turning point in my life. My self-esteem was soaring. I went to college in a great state of mind.

It is now seven years since my surgery, and I have a child of my own (that I successfully nursed). I hope that she will be happy with herself, but having "been there and done that," I know that I will do whatever it takes to increase her self-esteem—even if it means plastic surgery.

I would do it over again in a heartbeat.

—Jocelyn

desire for a quick fix to a social imperative. If the doctor is willing to put your teen's health and psychological well-being at risk for this type of procedure, he or she is not a good surgeon.

Again, do not consider surgically augmenting breasts until after the age of 18 unless there is an issue of minimal or no breast development or an issue of asymmetry with psychological implications. Dr. Richard D'Amico, a past president of the American Society for Plastic Surgeons, said in a position paper on breast implants, "It is important to get the message out to the media that there is a distinction between breast augmentation for purely cosmetic enhancement and those in need for more serious conditions."

When it comes to breast augmentation for teens, I have no one particular modus operandi. I have denied patients, deferred patients, and operated on patients (those with severely underdeveloped breasts). This topic is emotionally charged and receives much press—almost always the cases of botched teen plastic surgery you hear about in the media are related to breast augmentations.

For teenage girls, breast development is synonymous with femininity. As a physician, I must be sensitive to this. In cases of minimal or no breast development, sympathetic dialogue with both the teen and her parents is critical. The teen's feelings of inadequacy or not fitting in when she has absolutely no breast development should not be dismissed or trivialized. But implant surgery is a serious step that should not be considered lightly. I try to find out what the teen is looking for. If she brings in pictures of voluptuous celebrities, she raises a red flag. If she merely wants to feel feminine, a yellow light flashes and the discussion proceeds with caution.

> Almost always, the cases of botched teen plastic surgery you hear about in the media are related to breast augmentations.

Before the parents and I can decide to go forward with the surgery, I do not want any room for doubt that the teen's psychological well-being is affected by her lack of normal breast development. I must be convinced that the emotional need is in balance with the physical problem, and the patient must share my goal to create breasts of average size for her height, weight, body frame, and age.

If the teen, her parents, and I decide to green light a surgical solution, we can discuss the procedure in more detail. In thin girls, the silicone implant will, in my opinion, provide the best feel. In girls with more body mass, the saline implant is a good choice. At the time of this publication, there is a significant cost difference between the two types (silicone being more than twice the cost of saline), so that may factor into the decision. Placement of the implants—above or below the muscle— is up to the surgeon and patient. The location of incisions—underneath the breast, around the nipple, or in the armpit—also depends on the preferences of the surgeon and patient. There are no absolutes, though I do advise avoiding the belly button as a point of incision. This method, called transumbilical breast augmentation (TUBA), avoids breast incisions but makes it impossible to revise a breast without ultimately making an incision on the breast.

The patient must agree to allow enough time for recovery. As I've mentioned before, I prefer to time the surgery between high school and college, if possible. She must also commit to follow-up exams and proper maintenance. Implants do not last forever and must be managed and maintained for the life of the patient. As mentioned in the previous section, the implants may have to be repositioned, changed, or removed later.

If silicone implants are used, the FDA and the American Society of Plastic Surgeons mandate an MRI examination every three years. This is a good idea regardless of whether the implants are silicone or saline because an MRI has the ability to subtract away the implant and allow an excellent view of the breast tissue. Families need to be aware of this responsibility and the fact that their insurance company will probably not cover the cost of this mandatory exam.

Nipple Concerns: Inversion, Piercings, and Oversized Nipples

Stylistically, nipples have never been more prominent. Ever since women took off their bras in the '60s, the projecting nipple has been a fashion statement—an expression of sexuality, excitement, and youth. Even store mannequins now have nipples!

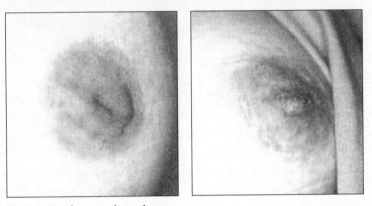

Correction of inverted nipple.

Inverted Nipples

Sometimes, however, a girl's nipple points in rather than out. This is called an inverted nipple. It can create psychological problems for teens, especially older teens entering into the world of sexual experiences. The problem also has potential ramifications later in life for breast-feeding and cancer detection. An inverted nipple can be easily corrected to the appropriate "out" position using local anesthesia in an outpatient setting.

Throughout my adolescent years I was self-conscious about my inverted nipples. They made my breasts look abnormal. I was going off to college and was stressing about this "deformity." In spite of what my pediatrician said, it bothered me. When my mother met a plastic surgeon who said it was a common problem with a simple solution, I was elated. How many years did I stress needlessly? I immediately went to have the procedure. It was indeed simple—I left for college two days later with a smile on my face.

—Betsy age 18

My daughter had inverted nipples as a child. As she approached her teen years it became a concern to her. As a dutiful parent I questioned my pediatrician; he said nothing could be done to correct it, and it was harmless. I trusted the doctor and pursued it no further, until the summer before college when I discovered just how emotionally bothered she was. By happenstance I met a plastic surgeon and related the situation to him. I'll never forget what he said. "Of course it's correctable! It is a small procedure under local anesthesia done right in the office." It was quick and painless, and it made my daughter feel wonderful as she embarked on her new college adventure.

—Sandra (mother)

Piercings and Large Nipples

It may be hard for parents to understand why on earth a teen (girl or boy) would want to pierce a nipple. A pierced nipple can stretch or tear—something that is definitely not a good fashion statement. Scarred nipples could present breast-feeding problems for future moms. Whatever his or her reason may have been for piercing a nipple, your teen doesn't have to live with that decision. Undoing it is simple (and, in fact, most

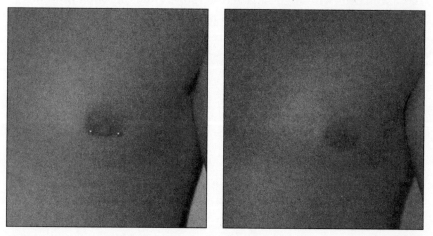

Correction of a nipple deformity from piercing, with removal of the bar, closure of the hole, and reconstruction of the stretched nipple.

likely less painful than getting the piercing). A pierced nipple can usually be corrected in the plastic surgeon's office under local anesthesia.

Likewise, teens with very big nipples (often called "silver dollar nipples") can opt for a nipple-reduction surgery. This is usually an in-office procedure. As with breast-reduction surgery, it does carry the small but possible risk of an inability to breast-feed.

Final Thoughts

To sum up:

- Breast reductions for female and male teens have a high rate of satisfaction and often make major improvements in quality of life: a win/win scenario.
- Breast augmentations in teens should never be considered unless there is a major psychological or physical issue related to asymmetry or underdevelopment. Tread cautiously in this area, and make sure you are working with an ethical plastic surgeon.
- Breast-feeding is safe and possible after breast augmentation and usually possible following breast reduction.
- Small surgical changes like converting an inverted nipple to an outward one or repairing damage from piercings are low-risk scenarios with high satisfaction rates. They can often be done as outpatient procedures in a plastic surgeon's office, where the necessary medical facilities are on-site.
- Mammograms may be done as the teen ages without worry.

10

Body Contouring

FINGERTIP FACTS

☞ Teenage obesity is now considered an epidemic.

☞ Massive weight loss in teens has major plastic surgical implications.

☞ Procedures to recontour the body involve large incisions and scars.

☞ Teens who need to lose large amounts of weight should seek a team approach.

☞ The readjustment for the teen who has lost a lot of weight is both psychological and physical.

☞ Body contouring surgery after weight loss is often not covered by insurance.

N AN IDEAL WORLD, this chapter would not have to be written, but in the real world, it must be written. It is a cautionary message as well as an informational one. Teenage obesity has become so prevalent that significant time, effort, and monies are being exhausted to treat the manifestations and subsequent side effects for a preventable situation.

Although I am a plastic surgeon, I am a physician first. I want all my patients to be healthy and happy. I want teens and families to do what is appropriate when it is appropriate. If they do not need surgery, they should not have it. If there are alternatives, they should be considered before surgery.

Until recently, teen plastic surgery has largely centered on structural issues that are out of the patient's control—such as problems with one's nose, ears, and breasts—and the psychosocial impact imparted by them. However, there is a new and rapidly growing area of plastic surgery that teens are being exposed to: body contouring after massive weight loss. Teens must now deal with surgical procedures that used to be reserved for adults—body lifts, abdominoplasties (tummy tucks), breast lifts, and arm and thigh lifts.

Young minds, with their desire for quick fixes, may not be able to truly understand the ramifications of body contouring and the scars that remain. This is a very complex issue with many layers—physical, emotional, and financial. This is why this chapter also serves as a warning for parents of young teens and adolescents: *Be proactive, so as to help prevent these surgeries from ever becoming necessary.*

In this chapter, I bring to attention the surgical treatments for obesity and their aftermath as well as the occasional situations in which liposuction may be justified. I also touch on other weight issues, including body dysmorphic disorder (BDD) and anorexia and bulimia.

Adolescent Obesity: Too Much TV, Not Enough PE

Recent studies out of major medical centers have confirmed what we already know from media blitzes and the increases in diet and exercise infomercials—adolescent obesity is on the rise. According to statistics released by the United States Department of Health and Human Services, 15 percent of all adolescents are considered markedly overweight, which is roughly 9 million teens in America alone. Four percent are considered morbidly obese, meaning they are at least one hundred pounds above ideal body weight.

With obesity comes the potential for significant medical problems: arteriosclerosis (hardening of the arteries with attendant heart and kidney disease and stroke), colon diseases including cancer, type 2 diabetes, polycystic ovary syndrome (in girls), hypogonadism (in boys), liver and gall bladder problems, and asthma and sleep apnea. Other physical problems include sanitary issues of sweating and rashes in the folds of the skin.

Until recently, teens with high blood pressure, heart disease, and diabetes were a rarity. It took decades of dietary abuse and lack of exercise for individuals to succumb to these ailments. Now they are approaching epidemic proportions in adolescents—a population that traditionally has been the healthiest and most active. Modern culture and its conveniences and advances (like TVs with remote controls, driving everywhere rather than walking, and spending hours in front of a computer) have left us with children suffering from diseases that stem from abundance.

Many teens are confronting not only the physical hardships of obesity but also its social implications and psychological ramifications. Obesity has a major emotional impact. Poor self-esteem, social isolation, and restricted quality of life have resulted in significant depression in many obese adolescents.

The Fight against Fat

This is not a diet and exercise book, nor is it a treatise on behavior modification. It is, however, a book about how surgery can impact upon a teen's well-being. Parents and children should know what may be in store for them if the path of obesity continues. Parents should also consider ways they can stop the situation from getting out of control in the first place.

National attention to the problem of obesity has led to significant efforts to stop its spread and to treat the afflicted. Many of the major weight-loss enterprises have developed programs for adolescents, and schools are reevaluating their meal and exercise programs. Even McDonald's has been pressured to create menu items without trans fats and has discontinued its "Super Size" options.

Centers of Excellence

Bariatric Centers of Excellence are institutions that use a team approach to guide patients and their families through organized and regimented weight loss, which could include bariatric surgery. The plastic surgeons on the team can explain the aftermath of massive weight loss and the possible need for re-draping surgeries. They can outline the options for body contouring and allow for advanced planning. The nutritionists on the team give weight-loss counseling, and the psychologists help the teen deal with his or her body-image issues both before and after the weight loss and the surgeries.

Major medical centers in your area can help you find a bariatric center of excellence that's right for your teen. For more information on the American Society for Metabolic and Bariatric Surgery and Bariatric Centers of Excellence, see the Resource Guide at the back of the book.

While these efforts are to be applauded, there is much we can do as parents on the homefront. Parental guidance and role modeling should be the first and foremost in the battle to regain teen vitality. This can no longer be a "do what I say and not what I do" situation. There are too many temptations in the fast food world to allow for choices without education. And education must begin early and be continual. Parents must lead by example. You cannot eat a Whopper and tell your kids to go to the salad bar.

> Parental guidance and role modeling should be first and foremost in the battle to regain teen vitality. This can no longer be a "do what I say and not what I do" situation. As parents, you cannot eat a Whopper and tell your kids to go to the salad bar.

After exhibiting healthy eating habits yourself as a role model for your teenagers, your next step of care is helping them make similar choices for themselves. Behavior modification is crucial to fighting weight problems. It is well known that diets have a history of failure. In fact, a conclusion from the February 2000 "Great Nutrition Debate" sponsored by the United States Department of Agriculture in Washington, DC, was that "diets" don't work. Yet many people buy in to the huge number of diet programs, books, and commercials touting successes only to find that they have wasted their money on false hopes and hype. A lifestyle change, not a fad diet, is in order. What works for losing weight is taking less fuel in and putting more energy out. Once a person has realized there must be a lasting change, then organized weight loss and exercise programs can be useful and beneficial.

Unfortunately, many teens in this instant gratification culture cannot control themselves and lack support systems to motivate restraint. If this is the case, they should be referred by their pediatricians to a bariatric center (preferably one that has been designated a "Center of Excellence" by the American Society for Metabolic and Bariatric Surgery) that deals with adolescent weight issues. These clinics can provide medications to curb appetites as well as psychological support. In certain individuals these programs may not yield results; those will need the next level of care—bariatric surgery.

Weight–loss Surgery: A Last Resort

Uncontrollable obesity has reached such dramatic levels that 200,000 or more surgical weight-loss procedures are now performed each year. The patients are primarily adults who are so overweight and have so many other weight-related medical issues that this is their best and last chance for success. They are selected carefully, as the risks for such surgeries are high, and drastic postsurgical lifestyle changes are mandatory.

The last fifty years of performing bariatric surgery on adults have given surgeons experience they can apply to bariatric surgery for teens and adolescents. Teen bariatric surgeries are being carefully monitored and assessed by the Teen-Longitudinal Assessment of Bariatric Surgery (Teen-LABS), an ancillary study of the Longitudinal Assessment of Bariatric Surgery (www.niddkLABS.org), sponsored and funded by the National Institute of Health. The number of bariatric surgeries for adolescents has increased threefold over the last decade, now making it approximately 1 percent of total weight-loss surgeries. This number will rise as the safety and efficacy of the procedures is confirmed.

Qualifications for Bariatric Surgery

The following indications must be present for a teen to be considered for bariatric surgery:

- Morbid obesity—usually overweight by at least one hundred pounds with an attendant increased risk for medical problems related to obesity
- Failure of behavior modification trials, including medications and psychotherapy
- Willingness to comply with long-term nutritional management program
- Medical and psychological justifications and clearances

Gastric Bypass versus the LAP-BAND Procedure

Bariatric surgery has taken on two forms: gastric bypass and gastric banding.

The bypass, which is a true surgical procedure, is the gold standard in weight-loss surgery to which results of alternative procedures will be compared. Gastric bypass surgery (GBPS) involves short-circuiting part of the stomach and small intestine to limit the amount and absorption of food. This surgery has a high success rate but also can have a high complication rate and requires long-term nutritional counseling to prevent vitamin and nutrient deficiencies that stem from the alterations.

A less-invasive procedure is gaining popularity in Centers of Excellence weight-loss studies: the LAP–BAND procedure. Here, an adjustable tube (band) is placed around the stomach through a small incision using laparoscopic techniques. The tube is regulated with a valve beneath the skin and can be loosened or tightened as needed. This serves to restrict volumes of food ingested. Although this procedure holds promise, it is too early to draw final conclusions. Potential drawbacks are the ability to cheat the system with liquids and problems with the device itself, especially over the long term.

The Lasting Legacy of Massive Weight Loss

Whether it was through surgery, exercise, a strict diet, or some other means, many teens have succeeded in losing weight. The overall benefit to society will not be known for decades, but the individual benefits physically and emotionally are undeniable—unless the teen suffers from the aesthetic problems of massive weight loss.

The downside of massive weight loss is that there is no guarantee that the teen's skin (referred to as the "envelope" among plastic surgeons) will respond kindly to the reduced contents—the loss of fat. Thinner does not necessarily mean tighter.

Teens who have lost a significant amount of weight, whether on their own with diet and exercise or with bariatric surgery, can find themselves with major aesthetic concerns, which can be isolated to one area or more global. There is no way to know before losing weight if the skin envelope will respond favorably. When it does not, teens can face all the problems older individuals who have lost massive amounts of weight do: sagging breasts and butts, hanging abdomens, and floppy arms and thighs. These problems can persist despite the teen's considerable efforts in aerobic and weight-training programs.

> I would venture to say that if educational programs for adolescents revealed to them the potential cosmetic challenges—like loose hanging skin—they could face from obesity even after weight loss, it would go a long way to be a visual reminder to eat less and exercise more.

Significant sagging skin can be as psychologically devastating to a fragile teen as being overweight and may cause some teens to consider "filling out" again.

(I would venture to say that if educational programs for adolescents revealed to them the potential cosmetic challenges—like loose hanging skin—they could face from obesity even after weight loss, it would go a long way to be a visual reminder to eat less and exercise more.)

Massive weight-loss patients find it hard to believe that their hard work of diet and exercise has left them short of their goals, which are primarily aesthetic. Even though they may be medically healthier, they view their success through the prism of how they look. From those trying to tighten up their loose skin, I constantly hear things like, "It's not fair. I go to the gym every day and do 300 sit-ups, and look at this belly!" or, "I lift weights, and yet my arms are like my grandmother's!"

Surgical improvements for the consequences of massive weight loss are available, but they are costly, are not always covered by insurance, and leave significant scars.

The good news is that surgical improvements for the consequences of massive weight loss are available, but bear in mind that they are costly, are not always covered by insurance, and leave significant scars.

BDD and Massive Weight Loss

Some weight-loss patients develop a unique type of body dysmorphic disorder; when this occurs, early psychologic intervention is very important. These teens see themselves as "fat forever" in spite of achieving satisfactory goals and, as a result, push their weight loss too far and become anorexic or bulimic. Others will try and pursue plastic surgery beyond what can reasonably be accomplished.

Surgery after Massive Weight Loss— Cutting, Darting, Pleating

As with other teen plastic surgeries, the surgeon must very carefully assess teens seeking surgery after massive weight loss. Like most teens, they want perfect results with little downtime and no risk, and their parents want no out-of-pocket expenses. Teens and families need to know of the complexities of body-contouring surgery, and they should have realistic expectations. There are bigger scars, more procedures, longer recoveries, and greater expenses than most people imagine. Many a patient, both adult and teen, has commented that losing the weight was easier than the later surgical transformations.

Any teen in the process of losing a significant amount of weight should probably have a consultation with a plastic surgeon to talk about body contouring. This way, the teen and family can learn ahead of time what happens to a body after the weight comes off. Once you and your teen are educated, you can plan for the surgery. Advanced financial preparation is especially important due to the high cost of these surgeries and if you want to attempt to receive coverage. Insurance companies are being flooded with claims involving this new type of reconstructive plastic surgery, and they are not forthcoming in providing coverage. They tend to view it as more cosmetic than functional or psychological.

If a problem is isolated to one body part, the surgery is more affordable and straightforward, and the results more predictable and accepted. When the problems are more global and the surgeries more extensive, issues can arise, and some potential patients simply can't afford the procedures. In fact, of the weight-loss patients studied at the University of Pittsburgh, 80 percent stated a desire for cosmetic body contouring, but only 12 percent actually went through with it. Their main reasons were costs for the procedures and time lost from school or work.

Teens who need surgery on more than a single anatomic part should seek out a Center of Excellence (see sidebar on page 156). These centers not only guide teens and their families through the weight loss and bariatric surgery but also through the staging and completion of redraping surgeries, which are discussed in the procedures section later in this chapter.

Questions to Ask

Is body-contouring surgery a possibility for your teen? Ask yourself the following questions:

1. **Has the weight loss been stable for at least one year?** This allows for nutritional stability and for the skin to shrink as much as possible.
2. **Is my teen otherwise in good health?** Careful medical management is crucial to avoid surgical complications—particularly problems with wound healing.
3. **Does my teen smoke?** Nicotine hinders healing and must be eliminated from the system at least six weeks before surgery.
4. **Is my teen psychologically prepared for the surgeries and recovery?** This process is arduous for patient and family.

5. **Do we all have realistic expectations?** Surgery will improve shape, but it cannot restore it to what it may have been without the weight gain.
6. **Are we prepared for the risks? Have we been informed?** Significant surgeries carry significant risks.

The Risks and Realities of the Surgery

Before a discussion can be undertaken regarding body-contouring surgical procedures, there must be time spent on the risks. Patients and their parents need to know that the procedures require a stay in the hospital and may in fact involve multiple surgeries (known as stages) over a few years. This should be discussed with the surgeon well in advance of the surgery so everyone understands and is on board with the process.

Because of the significant amount of skin to be removed, body-contouring surgery poses greater risks than standard cosmetic procedures. The patient spends more time on the operating table, especially when the surgeon is working on more than one area of the body. Prolonged anesthesia can mean longer recovery time and an increased risk of deep vein thrombosis (DVT), a blood clot commonly in the legs that could cause pulmonary embolism and even death. To prevent such catastrophes, many centers are anticoagulating (thinning the blood with medication) these types of patients. These treatments are state of the art but carry their own risks of excess bleeding, bruising, and delays in wound healing. It is a delicate balance to optimize these individuals.

Since the resections of skin are frequently big, drains—tubes to carry away any fluid accumulations under the skin—are usually used. Large incisions also mean larger wounds to heal and longer scars than one may imagine.

Many surgeons place their patients in support garments for the post-operative recovery period. These help hold the tissues in place and provide support and security to the patients.

Most procedures require hospital stays of between one and four days. Multiple-site surgeries require multiple incisions and cause more discomfort. For this reason, many surgeons opt for staged procedures (one area at a time) over a few years. This allows patients to recover physically, emotionally, and financially.

The Types of Procedures by Body Part

Different areas of the body require different procedures. The farther you go down the body, the more significant the deformity and the more difficult it is to correct. Let's look at each area from the top of the body to the bottom.

Face and Neck

Fortunately, even after significant weight loss, the face seems to be spared sagging. Face redraping procedures in teens are rare. Occasionally, a neck liposuction may be needed (see the section on liposuction later in the chapter).

Arms

With loss of volume, upper-arm skin can sag. Although this is bothersome, it is often a lesser priority in the treatment plans of body contouring in teens. However, sometimes a teen has so much hanging skin on his or her arms—known as "bat wings"—to make the surgery highly desirable. The surgery to fix this is called brachioplasty and it is done the same way on a teenager as it would be on an older individual. The procedure involves a long incision from the armpit (axilla) to the elbow. If the patient also has remaining excess fat, a spot liposuction may be added.

Breasts

Anything can happen with significant weight loss. It is possible for the breasts to reduce appropriately and become a nonissue. It is possible for them to shrink differently, resulting in size discrepancies. More often than not, the breasts sag and assume a much more elderly shape than a teen desires. Sagging breasts can be lifted (see chapter 10 for more details). Sometimes the patient has lost so much weight that lifting is not enough and she also needs an augmentation. Occasionally, in spite of weight loss, the breasts remain disproportionately large and require a reduction. Thus, the patient may need a lift, a reduction, an augmentation, or a combination of these, so the procedures must be tailored to the situation.

In patients who have lost an extreme amount of weight, the excess skin can go beyond the breast edge onto the flank and back. The surgeon can perform an extended procedure to include this excess skin, but this procedure will increase the length of the scars.

Teen boys also can be faced with sagging breasts after weight loss and may require excisional surgeries as well to tighten the chest area and create a more masculine physique.

Abdomen

This is the most common area for correction in the teen weight-loss patient. When abdominal girth recedes, a hanging curtain of skin (pannus) can remain. This is very frustrating because it cannot be disguised the way breasts can be in custom bras. Bathing suits and light clothing are difficult to wear, and self-esteem diminishes. No matter how many crunches the patient does in the gym, the pannus remains. Oftentimes, a patient and family will seek consultation, thinking that a minimal-scar liposuction will make it disappear. But only excision of the skin will resolve the problem.

There are two forms of excisional surgery for the surgeon and patient to consider for this situation: panniculectomy and abdominoplasty. In both procedures, the incision is large and extends from hip to hip across the front of the abdomen along the panty line. The goal is to redrape the front of the torso and, if needed, lift a sagging *mons pubis* (pubic area) as well.

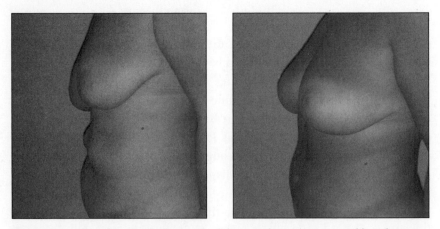

Body contouring after weight loss with abdominoplasty (tummy tuck) and mastopexy (breast lift) performed during the same surgery.

Panniculectomy removes the hanging curtain of skin, but it does nothing for the upper abdomen. It is a very useful procedure that can bring both cosmetic and functional relief from the rashes and irritations that often occur when the abdominal skin rubs against the pubic skin. Insurance companies will consider this for reimbursement if the patient can show documentation of dermatological problems (intertrigonal infections) in the pannus folds. The procedure is a direct excision of the curtain and involves no undermining (radical elevations) of skin. Healing is usually straightforward, and the complications are few. Panniculectomy helps to boost self-esteem and is a great first start for patients requiring multiple procedures.

Abdominoplasty is a "panniculectomy plus" procedure. The skin is pulled away up to the lower rib edges. The exposed abdominal muscles can then be tightened with sutures. Next, the skin is pulled down and the excess (the skin that hangs below the incision line) removed. The belly button is repositioned to a more youthful position as the skin curtain is resected. If a hernia is present, it can be repaired during the procedure.

Drains are used in both procedures, and both surgeries take between two and four hours under general anesthesia. Patients usually remain in the hospital for one day.

Liposuction may be used on the flank regions following the resections to smooth out the edges.

In some situations, the patient has lost so much weight that the horizontal incision is not enough and an up-and-down incision must be added. This fleur-de-lis pattern allows for even more skin to be removed, but it also adds a significant vertical scar that is hard to hide.

Thighs

As we move down the body, the severity of the sagging increases. Many weight-loss patients—despite hours of aerobics—suffer from loose skin on the inner thighs. This can be unattractive, and it also causes discomfort from continual rubbing.

A medial thigh lift removes the excess skin of the upper inner thigh. Incision patterns vary based on the deformity. Sometimes they are restricted to the groin creases, but other cases require an additional incision down the inside of the thigh from the groin to the knee.

Body Lifts

Some patients are physically, emotionally, and financially able to undergo multiple contouring procedures in one operation. These combinations are called body lifts. Figure 10.1 shows some of the areas that may be addressed with a body lift procedure.

Lower-body Lift

The lower-body lift procedure is more than an extended abdominoplasty or panniculectomy. Here the patient is turned over and the buttocks and thighs are lifted as well. It involves more time than abdominoplasty or panniculectomy alone, and the potential for complications increases as more is done. Recovery is also more arduous because a lower-body lift hinders walking and sitting in the very early recovery phase.

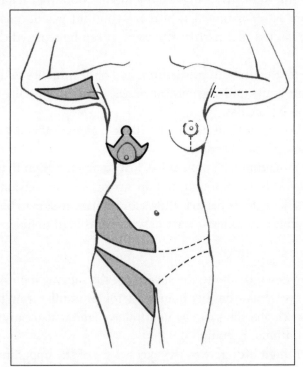

Figure 10.1 The excision patterns to remove excess skin and the scars that remain from the various body contouring surgeries.

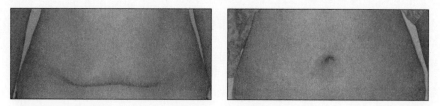

Abdominoplasty (tummy tuck) after weight loss.

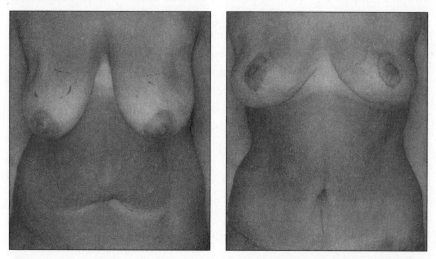

Abdominoplasty and mastopexy for body contouring following significant weight loss.

Upper-body Lift

An upper-body lift, which is a set of procedures, corrects the breasts and arms and extends onto the upper back to remove the rolls of excess skin there as well. Like the lower-body lift, this combination procedure takes longer and is more stressful for the patient in recovery than a single procedure.

Excisional body-contouring procedures can be very helpful to teens who feel miserable and trapped in their own skin after massive weight loss. The price is high in both cost and risks, but the rewards can be great. It is critical that a patient understands that incisions and scars are extensive, and that in general body-contouring surgery is not a quick fix. (I say in general because there are rare cases in which small weight losses have resulted in small but real deformities that can be handled singularly by one of the above individual procedures.)

Liposuction

Liposuction is the number-one plastic surgical procedure performed for cosmetic reasons in the world today. According to the American Society for Plastic Surgeon statistics, more than 250,000 liposuctions are done in the United States each year, representing nearly a quarter of all cosmetic surgeries. More than 4,000 of these were performed on teenagers.

One of the reasons for the liposuction's popularity is the minimal incision aspect. However, this can be misleading. Although the access sites are small, the spaces created to remove the fat are large. Furthermore, the smaller incisions do not mean fewer risks.

Liposuction should only be done on teens who have met the strictest of criteria. Many teens believe this to be the ideal quick-fix procedure with basically no incisions, and they may seek it as an easy weight-loss method. The surgeon and parents should make sure the teen is mature enough to understand that liposuction is surgery with risks.

> Liposuction is the number-one plastic surgical procedure performed for cosmetic reasons in the world today: More than 250,000 liposuctions are done in the United States each year, representing nearly a quarter of all cosmetic surgeries. More than 4,000 of these were performed on teenagers.

I will consider liposuction alone when isolated deposits of fat remain after a teen has normalized his or her body weight with a healthy diet and exercise program. Patients most often request my services for the outer thighs (the so-called "riding britches deformity") and under the neck. These are simple surgeries with rapid recoveries. Liposuction can also be used to supplement the excisional body-contouring methodologies described above when an area needs further refinement.

As with all surgery in teens, I must see that there is harmony between the physical need and the teen's emotional maturity to understand the risks as well as the benefits of surgery.

Final Thoughts

Parents should make a concerted effort to be proactive in preventing childhood obesity. This means leading by example with nutrition and exercise. This will go a long way in preventing the psychosocial and physical issues that confront many overweight adolescents.

If your child is significantly overweight consider researching out a center of excellence that focuses on weight loss. These centers involve many disciplines, including nutrition, medication, counseling, and surgery.

Those teens who have suffered from obesity and succeeded with massive weight loss may have to deal with the ramifications of a skin envelope that failed to shrink with their body. In these situations, body contouring surgery may be the only option to restore aesthetic balance and proportion. These are major surgical procedures that should be done by experts in the field of post-bariatric plastic surgery.

11

Skin

FINGERTIP FACTS

☞ The skin is the largest and most injury-prone part of the body.

☞ Scars can be improved but are never erased.

☞ The sun is not your skin's friend—exposure equals damage.

☞ Unwanted hair can be permanently removed.

☞ The secret to hair growth has yet to be unlocked.

☞ A new tattoo ink may help those with buyer's remorse.

THE SKIN IS PROBABLY the most traumatized part of a teen's body. Teens burn it, pierce it, ink it, shave it, and injure it in accidents. Youngsters may also be confronted with acne, acne scars, premature hair loss, and unwanted hair.

This chapter is not a treatise on dermatology or reconstructive plastic surgery on burns or other major skin deformities. Rather, it concerns itself with common teen skin issues that fall into the hands of a plastic surgeon: scars, tattoos, moles, piercings, and hair.

Teenage skin problems can be categorized into prevention and intervention. Many skin problems that teens suffer could have been avoided with forethought. A tattoo never has to be removed if it was never placed. There would never be an infection or a scar from a piercing if the piercing never occurred. Sun damage is a "buy now, pay later" phenomenon; premature aging and skin cancer are rarely seen early on, but the stage is set in the teen years.

When problems related to the skin occur, they can be emotionally devastating. Unsightly moles, unwanted hair, premature balding, post-acne scars, and scars from surgery or injury can elevate teen angst to new levels. And buyer's remorse can occur after a teen spontaneously decides to get a tattoo or piercing.

The Basics—Setting the Stage

The skin, as everybody knows, is the outer covering of the body. It is the body's largest organ and is the protective layer guarding the underlying tissues. The skin is the insulator, the temperature regulator, and the sensor. Skin is amazingly elastic and allows for movement and facial expression. Without a properly functioning skin envelope, it is impossible to survive. Just think of the movie *Goldfinger*. When the Bond girl is sprayed over every inch of her skin with gold paint, she suffocates. Her skin cannot "breathe," so she overheats and dies.

The skin has remarkable self-healing capability. Melanin absorbs the potentially harmful ultraviolet (UV) radiation from the sun, and the DNA-repair mechanisms in the skin may reverse some of that UV damage. Collagen, a basic building block of the skin, provides the scaffold for wound healing following injury. The aftermath of this repair process is called a scar—a small word for something that causes so much emotional havoc.

Skin has been classified on the basis of complexion and its susceptibility to damage from sunlight. These classifications serve as a useful barometer in assessing the likelihood of future problems, the ability of the skin to heal wounds, and what type of scars may be produced,

In 1975, Harvard dermatologist Dr. Thomas Fitzpatrick created a scale to assess skin and its tolerances. He broke it down into six types,

FITZPATRICK CLASSIFICATION SCALE

Skin Type	Skin Color	Characteristics
I	White; very fair; red or blond hair; blue eyes; freckles	Always burns, never tans
II	White; fair; red or blond hair; blue, hazel, or green eyes	Usually burns, tans with difficulty
III	Cream white; fair with any eye or hair color (very common skin type)	Sometimes mild burn, gradually tans
IV	Brown; typical Mediterranean Caucasian skin	Rarely burns, tans with ease
V	Dark brown; mid-Eastern skin types	Very rarely burns, tans very easily
VI	Black	Never burns, tans very easily

now called the Fitzpatrick Classification Scale. This scale helps all practitioners who work with skin to predict responses to damage.

By noting where your teen falls on this chart, you can see how prone he or she is to the damaging effects of the sun and how necessary protection from UV rays is—solar or salon. Knowing your child's skin type also provides you with insight into how red, dark, thick, or thin a scar may be (see the section on tanning and scars later in the chapter).

The skin is a surface as well as a barrier. As such, it is a host to many microorganisms, such as bacteria. Most times, these bacteria live in balance with the skin. Poor skin hygiene, however, can upset the skin's normal balance and lead to problems such as acne and infections. Oily skin is more prone to blemishes because the excess oil clogs the pores, facilitating the growth of bacteria, leading to "pimples." But this lubricant has a plus side in that it protects the skin from premature aging and wrinkles and keeps the skin smooth and moist.

There is an entire industry based upon keeping the skin clean and its moisture in balance. Dermatologists and aestheticians are specialists on skin health and treating problems such as acne. I will leave that to them, though I do provide in this chapter basic steps in daily skin care and discuss skin issues that require a plastic surgeon: removals and reconstructions.

Scars

Probably the two most common questions I am asked as a plastic surgeon are "Will there be a scar?" and "Can you remove this scar?"

There is an impression that plastic surgeons have a secret for dealing with scars that others do not. I have heard this misconception thousands of times in thousands of ways: "I thought plastic surgeons do scarless surgery," or, "My child wants to be a model. I need this scar removed!" or, "I cannot believe there is a scar. I thought you were a plastic surgeon." It's never that easy. Read on, and you'll see why.

What Is a Scar?

A scar is the result of an injury. It is part of the normal process of wound healing. Scars are made up of the fibrous, nonelastic tissue that replaces the normal elastic skin. Except in the case of the most minor and superficial of injuries, a violation of the integrity of the skin leads to some variation of scar formation.

> Younger people heal better; their collagen mechanism is superb. Unfortunately, this leads to more pronounced scars. Older individuals have weaker collagen-repair systems; this prolongs wound healing, but it leaves fainter scars.

The deeper the "insult" through the layers of the skin, the greater the need for biologic repair and the more likely the presence of a scar. The skin can't differentiate between a surgical cut and an accidental injury. It just knows it needs to repair itself for protection from the outside environment. What can be variable is the skin's response to the injury. Different parts of the body have different skin thickness and elasticity, which affects how a scar manifests. Activity and motion also affect healing. Genetics, too, play a part in scarring. No two people scar exactly the same way.

How Is a Scar Made?

As mentioned previously, collagen is the basic building block of skin tissue. It exists in very organized, linear patterns. When injury occurs, the repair process involves a "laying down" of new collagen. This pattern is less organized in the beginning, accounting for the initial thickness and redness. As the wound matures, the collagen becomes more organized, and the scar improves.

Younger people heal better; their collagen mechanism is superb. Unfortunately, this leads to more pronounced scars. Older individuals have weaker collagen-repair systems; this prolongs wound healing, but it leaves fainter scars.

There are also genetic components to scar formation. Research is ongoing to try to unlock these genetic secrets and find a way to manipulate wound healing and produce healthy repair with less scaring.

Why Are Some Scars Less Noticeable than Others?

There are a variety of factors that contribute to scar formation: depth of injury, type of skin, location of injury, and genetic predisposition to healing. The study of scarring is a treatise unto itself and is beyond the scope of any lay book. However, understanding certain basic facts about scarring can help teens and parents cope with the distress of scars and allow for intelligent decision making in improving and ultimately accepting scars.

- *Depth of injury.* Superficial traumas such as abrasions, scratches, and mild sunburns often heal without significant residual damage, and there is minimal—if any—scarring. The deeper the cut or the burn, the more wound healing and the more pronounced the scar. Because scars are stiff and inelastic, they often feel tight. Some scars, like the ones teens get from acne, can be depressed and pitted—so-called "ice pick" scars. Depressed scars also can result from trauma and other skin conditions like chicken pox. Finally, some scars can be thin and stretched (striae) and result not from external trauma but from sudden internal stretching; these are the stretch marks often seen with adolescent growth spurts and from sudden weight loss or gain.
- *Type of skin.* Different skin types respond differently to injury. Older, thin skin with weak collagen makes a weaker and softer scar. Younger skin with strong healing mechanisms makes significant scars that take time to mature and soften and fade. Fair complexions (those lower on the Fitzpatrick Classification Scale)

175

make lighter scars; however, one exception to this rule are people with red hair, whose skin will make a very red scar that takes a long time to fade. Darker complexions have thicker skin components with more oils and can make darker and thicker scars.

- *Location of injury.* The site of the injury can define the character of the scar. Wounds heal better when they are in "relaxed skin tension lines" (RSTL). The RSTL are generally perpendicular to the muscles beneath. All you have to do is animate your face and look at the folds and wrinkles to see where the favorable lines are. In the trunk and extremities, it is more complicated because there are many overlapping muscles. The skin pulls in many directions, limiting our ability to plan or predict wound healing.
- *Genetics.* Most scars heal in predictable ways based on the genetic makeup of the individual. If you heal favorably, you will make better (less obvious) scars. It is encoded in your DNA. However, different areas of the body heal differently. Just because you make a "good scar" on your face doesn't mean a scar elsewhere on your body will be the same.

There are two types of scars that are more problematic than normal scars because they result when the skin deviates from the normal wound-healing process. These are hypertrophic scars and keloids. A hypertrophic scar is an overresponse to wound healing in which the scar remains within the dimensions of the injury but can stay thick and red for a prolonged period of time—even years. A keloid is a variant of this excess collagen production that grows out of control, often extending beyond the borders of the initial injury. In this case, the collagen maturing system is failing to keep pace with excess collagen manufacturing. Hypertrophic scars and keloids can occur on anyone but are more prone in dark-skinned individuals and in areas such as earlobes, the chest, the back, and shoulders.

Treatments to Improve Scars

All scars are permanent—a word no teen or parent wants to hear. Until research reveals new ways to influence the way wounds heal, we are limited in what we can do for scars cosmetically. Plastic surgeons cannot do scarless surgery and cannot erase existing scars. For surgeons, this means an honest yet compassionate discussion with the patient about wounds and healing. The word "scar" has many negative connotations and psychological implications. Where surgeons accept it as part of the job, patients often see it as a constant reminder of the event—whether accident or surgery, elective or emergency.

Most scars will fade and blend into the background of the skin over time. But anxious teens and parents are always asking for "scar removal" treatments. Although no treatment will completely erase a scar, there are resources available to improve scars resistant to normal healing and fading and to help patients who want to be proactive and participate in the healing process.

> Plastic surgeons cannot do scarless surgery and cannot erase existing scars.

Scar revisions. Many times the problem is with the way the wound was initially repaired or healed. Scars can be irregular because of poor surgical techniques or because injuries healed without any repair at all. In these situations, cutting out the scar to re-create the initial wound followed by a proper reconstruction can improve the result.

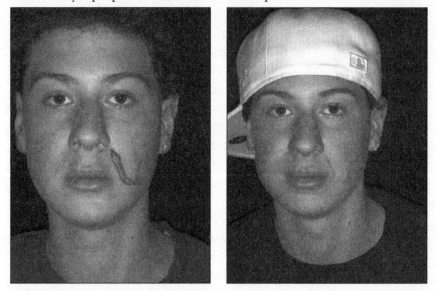

Hypertophic scar on left cheek with design for removal and reconstruction. Result after scar revision.

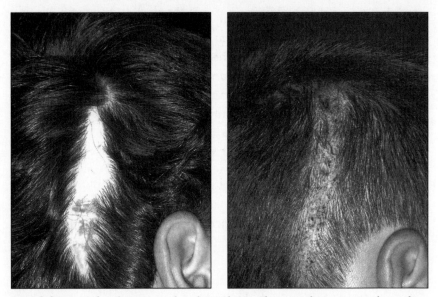

Scar deformity of scalp corrected with W-plasty. The inter digitation in the scalp tissues will prevent spreading and keep the hairs close together.

In some situations, a scar can be "rearranged" to change its direction so part or all of it falls within the RSTL. These so-called Z-plasties and W–plasties, which involve zigzag cuts for anti-tension rather than straight lines, can also release tight scars and allow for better healing. Sometimes a scar will actually be made larger to fit into the RSTL. Although longer, the new scar will heal in a less pronounced way.

Pressure and massage. It is well known that pressure placed on a healing scar may influence the blood flow into that scar and allow it to flatten and soften. For body and extremity scars, pressure garments can be custom made to provide appropriate amounts of pressure on a continual basis. For facial scars, this is not practical, so frequent massage is often recommended.

Vitamin E. Almost in the category of legend is the recommendation to use vitamin E on scars. This fat-soluble vitamin can penetrate the oily skin surface and weaken collagen. Many patients break open oral vitamin E capsules and rub them on the scar. It is hard to know if it is the vitamin or the massage that is helping. What we do know is that overindulging in vitamin E can weaken the surrounding tissues. (I had a patient who, without my knowledge, applied so much vitamin E to her healing breast-reduction incisions that she actually weakened the scars to the point of opening them.) It is best to speak to your treating physician before using vitamin E.

Silicone. Silicone placed over a scar creates a barrier of protection, allowing the healing tissues to retain moisture and provide gentle pressure. Silicone can be used as sheets placed over the incisions and early scars or as gels spread onto the scar.

Steroids. Steroids inhibit collagen repair and therefore wound healing. They can be applied to the scars topically as creams or as injections into hypertrophic scars and keloids. Steroids should not be used to treat normally healing scars, as they can weaken the wound and cause it to open.

Surface adjustments. Dermabrasion and laser resurfacing treatments have been used to smooth out scars and the surrounding skin. Other lasers can decrease the new circulation to the scar (neovascularization) and improve the overall healing.

Radiation therapy. Low-dose radiation is used as part of a treatment program to treat keloid scars when they fail to respond to more conservative measures such as pressure, steroids, and scar revision, and when they recur.

> Overindulging in vitamin E can weaken the surrounding tissues. I had a patient who, without my knowledge, applied so much vitamin E to her healing breast-reduction incisions that she actually weakened the scars to the point of opening them.

I now feel as though I can dress in a way a normal teenager would dress, because they no longer see my scar as me. They don't ask me questions like "What happened to you?" or "Why do you have a big scar on your chest?" My plastic surgery scar revision has allowed me to wear today's styles, including a two-piece bathing suit. Even though I knew the scar did not define me, others were using it as such. Now I feel much better about myself.
—Kathy, age 16

A Word on Lasers

The term LASER (light amplification by stimulated emission of radiation) has become a household word. But there is no single laser that practitioners use universally. Different lasers have different wavelengths and treat different problems. Vascular-specific lasers, such as the pulsed dye laser, can reduce the redness in a scar that results from increased blood circulation in the micro-structure of the scar. These lasers can also be helpful in treating some stretch marks with discoloration. Ablative lasers can smooth down irregularities from post-acne scarring. There are nonablative, or fractional, lasers that can tighten skin, reduce pore size, and improve stretch marks. Laser technology is constantly changing. By the time you finish this book, "old" lasers will probably have been replaced by ones we are not even aware of now!

For more information on lasers, refer to the resource guide at the back of the book.

Combination therapies. The demand to improve scars is so high that the industry has responded by manufacturing products that combine the silicone gel, vitamin E, and steroids (as well as other homeopathic remedies such as onion extract). Although they are available over the counter in pharmacies, I personally do not recommend you use them without your surgeon's knowledge. Patients who choose over-the-counter remedies like these need to be monitored closely to ensure that the treatment is not in fact causing harm.

> As a parent of a child who had had major surgery, I was grateful for her health. I was not really concerned about the cosmetics of her scar. I thought it was inconsequential. I soon realized it was not the case for her. Kathy had grown tired of people asking her "What happened?" Even a simple explanation would bring on more questions. The last straw was when a store clerk embarrassed her in public with her inquisitiveness. Kathy wanted the scar improved. The surgery made a tremendous difference in her outlook. The scar is not gone, but it has improved dramatically—along with Kathy's self image.
> —Rina (mother)

Intentional Scarring

In some cultures around the world, it is common for people to intentionally introduce wounds and scars as a form of decoration. Though this practice isn't a norm in Western societies, a person of any nationality can suffer from a psychological illness that causes him to want to self-mutilate by cutting his skin. People with this illness are frequent visitors to emergency rooms and often have extensive scars, usually on their extremities. A teen who is "cutting" needs to see a mental health practitioner and deal with the underlying issues. Once the psychological problem is under control, the teen can consider plastic surgical methods to diminish the physical result of their illness.

Scars from Acne and Chicken Pox

Many a teen has appeared in a plastic surgery or dermatology office distraught over the aftermath of chicken pox or acne. These afflictions damage the integrity of the skin and, in the worse cases, leave their marks.

Chicken pox often leaves depressed saucer-shaped scars. If a patient is bothered by these scars, there are techniques such as subcision that break up the tetherings and allow the scars to lift and flatten. In some instances, "filler" substances like hyaluronic acids can be injected into the subcised spaces to hold the lifting. Chemical peels and certain laser therapies can smooth the edges of scars for blending. A deep saucer can be traded for a linear scar within the relaxed skin tension lines. Sometimes a chicken pox scar will thicken and require excision and treatment like any other hypertrophic scar.

Acne can clear and leave no residual problem, or it can create havoc on the skin with many different patterns of scarring. There can be cysts that require removal by incision or excision and leave scars; there can be craters and pitted scars (ice pick scars); and there can be hypertrophic and even keloid scars. When a teen's acne has been resolved, scar revision treatments can be considered. There are many post–acne scar skin care techniques, including subcisions, direct excisions, dermabrasion, and laser treatments to smooth down the irregular surfaces left by the scarring.

An Ounce of Prevention...

Unfortunately, improvement of scars does not mean erasure. The best way to keep skin free of acne scarring is to prevent acne as much as possible.

Acne usually begins with puberty, when hormonal changes cause increases in oil production in the sweat glands. The oils can become trapped in the top, dead layer of the skin (keratin) and allow for bacterial growth (*P. acnes*). Dermatologists recommend first cleansing and decreasing the oil residues and the bacterial load in the skin's clogged pores. Next, patients should gently exfoliate to remove the keratin layer and then apply topical medications like benzoyl peroxide and antibiotics. Oral antibiotic therapy can be added if needed. Female patients can sometimes keep acne in check with certain birth control pills that help control hormones.

In very difficult cases, dermatologists will consider a photodynamic therapy known as "Laser and Levulan." For this treatment, the dermatologist applies to the skin a compound called alpha-aminolevulinic acid, which seeps into the pores. The doctor then uses a vascular laser to activate the compound, which attacks and kills the bacteria in the pores. Another laser-based therapy is photopneumatic therapy (Isolaz). This couples a vacuum to remove dirt from the pores and a laser to kill the bacteria. These are safe, effective measures that teens should try before resorting to isotretinoin (Accutane or Roaccutane). This drug is used only in the most refractory cases of acne. It works exceedingly well but carries risks. The patient may experience dry mouth and nail peeling from the decrease in oil production. The patient must also avoid intense sunlight and shouldn't have elective surgery for one year following the use of isotretinoin because of an increased risk of unfavorable scarring. Patients using isotretinoin must not get pregnant while undergoing treatment, because the medication also increases the risks of birth defects.

Acne can also arise from stress and can sometimes develop under surgical dressings like splints after rhinoplasty. When this type of acne occurs, treatment is usually basic and the resolution rapid.

Basic Skin Care Tips for Teens

PREP

- Prepare—cleanse with pH balanced, non-comedogenic products
- Renew—use retinol products to stimulate collagen daily
- Exfoliate—remove dry, old skin cells weekly
- Protect—use sun-protection products continually

Other Helpful Tips

- **Avoid smoking.** Nicotine damages the circulation to the skin and increases collagen breakdown.
- **Avoid excess ultraviolet ray exposure.** Use sun protection, and stay away from tanning beds.
- **Eat healthy, preservative-free foods, and drink lots of water to improve the pH balance in the skin.** Alkaline tissues fight the acidic free radicals that break down collagen.
- **Exercise.** Working out increases circulation to the skin and reduces stress.
- **Understand your skin type.** Not everyone needs a moisturizer.

Tanning: Buy Now, Pay Later—
The ABCs of Ultraviolet Radiation

What teen does not adore being at the beach or pool under the sun? Young and healthy teens with wrinkle- and blemish-free faces never believe that premature aging from excess and unprotected sun exposure will ever happen to them. Gone may be the days of sun reflectors and "baby oil and iodine," but the beach remains full of glistening bodies refusing to block out the sun. In fact, the teen sense of invincibility—the "I will never age" mindset—also takes teens to the tanning beds and salons, which are in fact more harmful.

This is not a call to live inside or go out only on cloudy days. Everyone needs some sun exposure. It is one of our primary sources of vitamin D for metabolism of calcium; remember those old TV ads, "Healthy bones with sunshine vitamin D"? Sunshine also feels good. It is wonderful to enjoy a sunny day. What is dangerous is unprotected overexposure to the sun's ultraviolet rays. Teens are the most vulnerable. Between sports and summer vacations, they are exposed to more than half of their lifetime dose of UV radiation.

UVA, UVB, and UVC are the three types of UV radiation emitted by the sun. Fortunately, clouds and the ozone layer provide some protection from their damaging effects. Even so, enough passes through to cause long-term damage to skin. UVB, the "burn ray," is responsible for the sunburn, which damages the superficial layers of the skin. UVA, the "aging ray," penetrates deeper into the skin and is responsible for both the suntan and the long-term damage to the skin. The third ray, UVC, does not make it to the Earth.

As harmful as sunning may be, tanning in salons is worse. The rays in tanning beds are primarily UVA, so they go deep into the skin. Traditional tanning beds can emit doses of UVA three times greater than those of the sun, and the newer high-pressure sun lamps can put out more than fifteen times the UVA and UVB of the sun. Tanning beds are of such concern that the World Health Organization called for teens to be banned from access to them without parental consent.

Skin contains a variable amount of a chemical called melanin, which is produced by cells called melanocytes. Melanin is the body's defense against the sun. The lighter the complexion, the less melanin, and vice versa. Darker complexions get darker in the sun, and lighter complexions may freckle or turn red.

A WORD OF CAUTION: Regardless of complexion, if a person has recently had surgery or sustained an injury, the sun will darken fresh scars and increase the time it takes them to heal and fade.

The other major line of defense is sunscreen. If your teen is out in the sun, use it and use it often!

As harmful as sunning may be, tanning in salons is worse. The rays in tanning beds are primarily UVA, so they go deep into the skin. Traditional tanning beds can emit doses of UVA three times greater than those of the sun, and the newer high-pressure sun lamps can put out more than fifteen times the UVA and UVB of the sun.

In 2008, more than 2.3 million teens visited tanning salons in the United States. A study reported in the *British Journal of Cancer* in 2000 and corroborated in the 2005 *Archives of Dermatology* confirmed that early and repeated UVA exposure from tanning beds increases the risk for some type of skin cancer in the future by 75 percent. These same studies revealed that using a tanning bed more than ten times in a year upped that risk ante by 800 percent for melanoma—the deadliest of skin cancers.

Tanning beds are of such concern that the World Health Organization called for teens to be banned from access to them without parental consent. The Food and Drug Administration (FDA), the Centers for Disease Control (CDC), and the American Academy of Dermatology have reiterated this warning and are trying to regulate the nonmedical use of tanning beds.

In response to these warnings, sunless, or "fake," tanning products have been developed and have become sophisticated enough to produce an effect similar to the real deal. These products, whether used at home or in salon spray booths, use the ingredients DHA (dihydroxyacetone) and erythrulose. These are not dyes, stains, or paints but harmless bio-chemical compounds that react with the cells on the skin's surface (the keratin layer) to create browning. The tan lasts about a week and then fades gradually as exfoliation occurs. There are also temporary bronzers that come in powders, sprays, mousses, gels, lotions, and moisturizers. They basically coat the skin with a "tan" that is washable and easily removed.

Most of the "fake" tans do not contain sunblocks, meaning they merely color the skin and don't protect against the sun. So teens should always apply sunblock on top of these tans when going out.

The take-home message for parents and teens is that there is no such thing as safe suntan indoors or outdoors. Remember:

1. If you want a tan, fake it and keep your skin intact.
2. Always use sunblock to avoid burning. Using sunblock as a regular part of skin care during the teen years is an investment in younger, healthier-looking skin later on in life.

Moles: Are They Really Beauty Marks?

Brown spots, or moles (also called nevi), on the body used to be called beauty marks, and some considered them fashionable. Most people have at least forty moles. Although a few may be present at birth, most appear during the teen years. Moles can be small and flat or large and raised. *It is important to acknowledge and act on moles that change.* Increases in size or changes in shape and/or color are signs of activity and can increase chances of progression to malignancy. Moles that exhibit these changes should be removed.

Some moles are in areas that are hard to see. Body checks by a dermatologist or pediatrician should be part of a teen's yearly checkup. If these exams reveal moles that have changed or are of aesthetic concern, your child's doctor should refer you to a plastic surgeon who can perform the necessary removal and reconstruction. Moles in areas of constant irritation—palms, soles, belt lines, bra lines, and beard lines—also should be

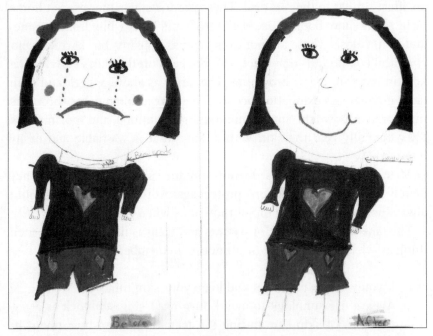

A 6-year-old girl with multiple moles on her neck. The "before" drawing shows her unhappiness with her big brown spots. After removal, she is happy and feels like the other children in her world.

186

removed. Continuous trauma can cause a mole to possibly change from benign to malignant.

Removing a Mole

Most teens seek mole removal not because of a disease but because of their unfavorable look. Some moles have unsightly hairs and can become centers of attention and embarrassment. A teenager with a mole in a prominent place might feel that people focus on the mole rather than on him or her. Dr. Erik Erikson, a famed child psychoanalyst, once reported on an adolescent who referred to himself as "the mole and me."

Most moles can be easily removed under local anesthesia in an office setting. The trade-off is a scar, although when the removal procedure is well planned and the incisions are well placed, the scar should fade into the skin lines.

Some moles are large; these require more advanced techniques for removal, such as staged serial excisions. First, the surgeon performs a partial excision, usually removing one-third to one-half of the mole (nevus), using local anesthesia. Once the wound has healed and the surrounding skin has relaxed—usually in about six weeks—the surgeon can remove what remains. This technique takes advantage of skin elasticity and allows for smaller overall incision lengths.

If a mole is very large and of significant medical concern, removal may require rotations of skin (known as flaps), or skin grafts, or even the use of tissue expanders to prestretch the adjacent skin to slide into the defect created by the excision. (These are complex procedures that are further explained in chapter 13.)

Every removed mole should be sent for biopsy! Malignancy, although uncommon in teens, can and does occur.

> I had a large "birthmark" on my face. It clouded the image I saw in the mirror. Maybe others did not mind it or care about it, but to me it was all I saw. I was 17 and about to go off to college. People come and go in your life, but you must face yourself for the long haul. I wanted a "clean start with a clean face." I was willing to trade a scar that would fade for the big brown spot on my face.
> —Devorah

Tattoos and Piercings: The Body as a Canvas

Teens are always in search of ways to express themselves. Tattoos and piercings are becoming a more common form of self-expression for people of all ages. Tattoos are no longer just for sailors, and earrings aren't relegated to the world of pirates. Body art has gone mainstream.

Everyone accepts pierced earlobes, and even infants can be seen with them. It is when piercings appear in unlikely places that parents' hearts skip a beat. I have seen nose, nipple, belly button, and vaginal labial rings on teens. I have seen posts in the ear cartilages, eyebrows, lips, and tongue. I have even seen a teen with safety-pin piercings across his neck. What a teen needs to know is that once they've pierced their body, the hole remains. Even if they remove the metal and the hole gets smaller, a small reminder will always be left behind. Especially large or problematic holes or scars may require surgical intervention, but surgery cannot repair every kind of piercing (see the procedures chapters in this book that relate to the body part affected).

Today, tattooing—or permanent body art—is pervasive. It is estimated that more than 10 million individuals have at least one tattoo. It has been estimated by the Pew Research Center and corroborated in a Harris poll that 50 percent of those who get tattoos regret their decision, and 20 percent try remedies for removal.

Past methods for tattoo removal were crude, with variable outcomes. Small ones could be surgically excised and traded for a scar. Larger ones were dermabraded (sanded) to expose the pigment and then treated with salt solutions to leach out the pigment. Often the discomfort from the treatment was worse than getting the tattoo and the results less attractive. Some tattoos cover such large portions of the skin that there is nothing to be done except learn to live with the decision.

Laser therapies have improved tattoo removal. They direct certain energy frequencies toward specific ink colors. The goal is to break up the ink particles into minute fragments that the body can then absorb. It is important to seek out a physician with the complete knowledge of lasers before considering this treatment. Some tattoos may be resistant to removal and will always leave a shadow. Furthermore, lasers in the wrong hands can create significant scarring.

There is hope for future fans of body art—and their distressed parents. Infinitink is a new tattoo ink that can be completely removed by laser therapies. Developed by Freedom2, the ink uses natural vegetable pigments stored in microcapsules, a technology the company calls Particle Encapsulation and Enhancement (P2E). Lasers can more easily disrupt these capsules and allow for the inks to dissolve. In essence, the tattoos are permanent until you no longer want them. This is a major breakthrough. The FDA does not regulate tattoo inks, and there can be health dangers in getting tattooed. Some inks are linked to cancer, and some can cause increased scarring and allergic reactions. If Infinitink passes the test of time, we can hope that all parlors will be mandated to use this type of technology.

Hair: Location, Location, Location

Baldness

Balding issues in teens are unusual, except for rare medical conditions beyond the scope of this book. Most male pattern balding doesn't begin until the man is in his 30s and slowly develops through his 40s. So if your teen, male or female, is showing signs of hair loss, a complete medical workup is necessary. Sometimes hair loss is temporary, brought on by stress or iron deficiencies. Thyroid issues can also affect hair growth, and some teens suffer from psychological illnesses that cause them to pull out their hair.

However, for the teen male whose genetics predispose him to baldness, premature thinning can be very distressing. Most often a teen seeks help because of a receding or thinning hairline. Although transplantation techniques have come a long way from the "doll's head" plug look, transplants are inappropriate for teen boys. The principle behind hair transplantation is to place hair follicles from the back of the scalp into the areas that are devoid or thin. When a balding pattern is defined, these operations can be planned to diminish the baldness. But the ultimate pattern of baldness cannot be predetermined in the teen years; therefore, it is difficult to plan where to take the hair from and where to put the hair.

Fortunately, there are other treatments these teen patients can consider. The two FDA-approved medicinal remedies to stave off or delay hair loss are minoxidil (Rogaine) and finasteride (Propecia).

Minoxidil was first used as a blood pressure medicine because it opens up blood vessels (vasodilation). Patients taking the drug noted hair growth, and researchers believe that this growth derived from increased circulation to the scalp. Minoxidil is now a topical solution available over the counter. Patients apply it directly to the scalp and must use it continually. Success is variable: a third of patients will grow hair, a third will get "peach fuzz," and the final third will see no change.

Finasteride is an inhibitor of the male hormone DHT, which induces baldness. It is an oral medication originally used to treat prostate disease in older men. A side effect (experienced by 2–4 percent of teens) is a decrease in sexual drive; this is restored when the drug is stopped.

A teen using either of these medications on a long-term basis should do so under the supervision of a dermatologist or a specialist in hair loss to monitor any possible side effects.

Genetic research is now ongoing to unlock the secrets behind baldness. The best future hope for those destined to be bald lies here.

Short hairstyles and shaved heads among celebrities have helped teens embrace heads without hair.

> As a young girl I grew up in the 60s and 70s with the problem of unwanted facial and body hair. Removal options were limited, painful, and worst of all temporary. Fortunately today, with laser technology, results are better, easier, and longer lasting. My daughter inherited my trait for "hirsuitism." I am glad she will not need to endure social angst or put up with the difficulties in removal.
> —Diane (mother of a teen girl)

Body Hair Be Gone

Unwanted hair can be very distressing, especially for girls. No female wants a beard or a mustache. Situations like this demand a medical workup to search for the root causes. Also, in this bikini-ready-body culture, men and women are seeking to remove most of their body hair.

In the past, hair removal meant waxing, shaving, or electrolysis. The first two are temporary; the latter is permanent but can be painful and leave small inflammations called folliculitis. Creams such as Vaniqa (eflornithine), which are designed to slow hair growth on the face, have been used with some success. But they do not permanently cure unwanted hair growth.

The advent of laser technology has revolutionized hair removal. Laser treatments are available that can significantly, if not completely, remove dark hair. (Laser light seeks the dark pigments.) Multiple treatment sessions are required because hair grows in three phases, and any one session only eradicates one-third of the volume—hair in the anagen, or growth, phase of the cycle. Treatments are relatively painless, but if they're performed in the wrong hands, they can lead to pigment changes and possibly scars. Individuals with suntans cannot have laser hair removal until the tan is gone, or they risk pigment changes to the skin. In the past, the ideal patient had dark hair and light skin. Now, even naturally dark-skinned individuals can benefit from laser treatments. At the time of this writing, blondes are not suitable candidates for laser therapies, but research is under way to develop treatments that are effective on light hair.

There are some light-therapy hair-removal systems now cleared by the FDA for home use on areas other than the face and genitals. Ask your dermatologist about these before trying them. Avoid unsupervised treatments, and try a test spot if you are unsure.

Final Thoughts

The skin is the most exposed and vulnerable organ in our body. Whether caused by nature or intention, skin problems, such as overexposure to the sun, piercings, tattoos, accidents, or surgery, can have lifelong ramifications and can only sometimes be repaired. Changes in moles, excess body hair in girls, and thinning hair in boys should be evaluated by a medical specialist such as a dermatologist or endocrinologist.

12

Ethnic Surgery: From Cultural Assimilation to a Culture of Beauty

FINGERTIP FACTS

☞ Twenty percent of all plastic surgery is performed on minority groups.

☞ Desires for cultural assimilation and anonymity have been re-placed by a desire for beauty.

☞ Teens' reasons for wanting change need to be assessed.

☞ Ethnic minority teens may see what they want but may not un-derstand the risks unique to them.

THE WORLD IS GETTING SMALLER and smaller day by day. No longer are cultures and people separated and isolated. Societies have blended, races have blended, and different ethnic groups are now a part of the melting pot that is the world today.

Plastic surgery has felt the impact of ethnic identity and is responding to the needs and desires of this clientele. Historically, plastic surgery was a means to eliminate perceived negative features in a minority patient to bring the patient closer to cultural anonymity. Today, as the melting pot is stirred, people have developed a composite view of beauty and want the best of all worlds. It is the culture of beauty that defines acceptance, not the culture of ethnicity. If there is a prejudice today, it is based on deviations from standards of beauty rather than race or national origin.

This chapter looks at how desires for surgery have changed through the generations. It also discusses the benefits, risks, and outcomes of surgery on people of different ethnic groups.

Ethnic Surgery: The Beginnings

"Ethnic surgery" is rooted in cultural assimilation and anonymity. The early American identity was that of the Northern Western European. Anyone who looked different was perceived as different and treated with prejudice. Plastic surgery quickly became "a way to change rather than cope and to alter rather than endure," according to Frances Cooke Macgregor in *Transformation and Identity: The Face and Plastic Surgery* (1974).

Early plastic surgical records are replete with cases of the Jewish nose, the Italian nose, and the Greek nose. This was the most identifiable feature of this immigrant group and was the first structure to change as they became Jewish Americans, Italian Americans, and Greek Americans. The entertainment industry reflected this change, as early vaudevillians tried to improve their limelight personas for the silver screen. One of the most famous examples is Fanny Brice, America's original "Funny Girl." In an attempt to elevate herself from the Ziegfeld Follies and create a more acceptable look for serious roles in the new era of movies, she underwent rhinoplasty in 1923. This trend continued, and notables such as Milton Berle and Dean Martin followed suit.

The next wave of plastic surgery for ethnic assimilation involved Asian war brides, for whom operations to Westernize the "Oriental eye" became popular. Literature of the time even describes many cases of American Army plastic surgeons operating on natives in the occupied

194

countries after World War II and the Korean War. This trend continued as African Americans tried to avoid the ravages of racial bigotry by intuitively following what Knight Dunlap wrote in his 1920 book *Personal Beauty and Racial Betterment*: "Beauty is a positive created by eliminating the negative—race, deformity and deviation from average." Thus, they attempted to whiten their skin, straighten their hair, and thin their noses.

Ethnic Surgery Today

The desire for ethnic assimilation and anonymity has faded today, as most individuals considering plastic surgery now want to improve their looks rather than drastically change them. People want to retain "clan identification" and remain bonded to their cultural families. The standards of the day are driven by ideals of beauty, as opposed to ethnic erasure, and, as Lois Banner writes in *American Beauty* (1983), "American ideals of beauty have become a composite over time—melting-pot beauty." Beauty is no longer synonymous with solely "white" features. Think

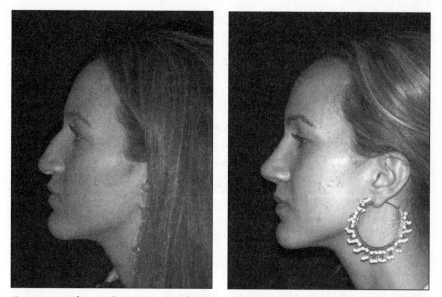

Correction of an "ethnic" nasal deformity consisting of a large bump and a drooping tip. Rhinoplasty reestablishes facial balance and harmony."

of Mick Jagger's and Angelina Jolie's full lips—features that were once considered undesirable African American traits. They are now a commonly accepted and sought after standard of beauty.

As minorities take their place in the melting-pot society, they are no longer viewed as self-hating or rejecting their roots if they seek to improve their looks with plastic surgery. And in fact, they're doing just that. In 2008, despite an overall 2 percent decline in cosmetic surgery procedures, the number of Hispanics who underwent plastic surgery increased by 18 percent, the number of Asians by 5 percent, and the number of African Americans by 10 percent—totaling more than 3 million surgeries. Since 2000, surgery on ethnic minorities has increased 215 percent. The current trend is for individuals to cherry-pick enviable features and request surgery for them. Beauty has become a hybrid mix—people want the best of everything!

> The current trend is for individuals to cherry-pick enviable features and request surgery for them.

Ethnic Surgical Preferences

Middle Eastern/Mediterranean: Rhinoplasty

People of Middle Eastern descent can have very defining noses. They not only are large by Western standards, but they can often have drooping nasal tips. Rhinoplasty to decrease the size of the nose and elevate the tip is one of the most sought-after procedures for this ethnic group. This desire for refinement is not limited to Middle Easterners in America; rhinoplasty is the number-one plastic surgical procedure in Iran today. More nose jobs are performed there than anywhere else in the world.

Asian: Blepharoplasty (Eyelid Surgery), Rhinoplasty, Breast Augmentation

Traditionally, Asian features consist of slight bodies with small breasts and distinctive eyes. The eyes are unique because they have what is called a single lid with a fold that extends into the inside corner of the eye. These hallmarks have changed in some individuals as intermarriage has hybridized looks. Other Asian individuals desire that melting-pot appearance and seek out surgical correction.

Many Asian noses are flat, lacking bony height in the bridge. Surgery to refine this involves the addition of structural support in the form of bone and cartilage. These tissues are "borrowed" from the nasal septum, the ear, the rib, and/or the hip. They are onlayed to create a stronger, more projected nose.

Breasts, as discussed in a previous chapter, are often viewed as *sine qua non*—essential—to femininity. Many females of Asian descent have seen friends who, either by nature or surgery, are more endowed, and as they move further away from their roots, the desire for larger breasts increases. One of the most popular operations for Asian women is breast augmentation.

Although Westerners are fascinated with the allure of the "Asian eye," many Asians seek a more Occidental look with a double lid. The necessary surgery is a variant of the cosmetic blepharoplasty, in which the surgeon repositions the skin of the upper lid at a higher level to reveal a rim that can accommodate makeup. This procedure also pushes back some of the bulging upper eyelid fat to further define the eye anatomy.

African American: Breast Reduction, Nasal Augmentation, Chin and Jaw Surgery

Features on black individuals can vary based on their background. The black and white races have mixed for long enough that many blended features are now part of their genetic makeup. Once, mixed individuals were ostracized, but now many are adored for their refined appearance. Subsequently, there has been an increase in Americans of black heritage seeking surgery for certain features.

Many black women are very well endowed in the breast area and desire a proportional correction. The breast-reduction procedure is the same as for all other individuals with macromastia, except that the patient and surgeon must consider the possibility of increased scarring, as some black individuals have a tendency toward hypertrophic scars and keloids.

Part of the genetic structure of a person of African descent can be a flatter, broader nose, a prominent upper jaw, and a smaller lower jaw. If a patient desires surgical alteration of these features, he'll generally need orthognathic surgery to reposition the upper and lower face in conjunction with orthodonture (braces). Patients who don't want such extensive surgery have opted for chin and nasal augmentation. The chin is advanced as discussed in chapter 7. The nose requires similar techniques to those of the Asian nose, in which the projection is increased to create the illusion of a narrower base. Wide nostrils are narrowed to complete the look.

Hispanic: Breast Augmentation, Liposuction, Nasal Surgery

The latest ethnic group to enter the arena of plastic surgery has become the most prevalent. The goals of Hispanic patients are diverse. Many seek body contouring to augment the top and reduce the bottom. Breast augmentation and liposuction are two of the most popular procedures. Additionally, many seek out nasal surgery to create a more refined profile.

Ethnic Surgery and Teens

Many teens of diverse ethnic backgrounds have become "Americanized" socially and, like all impressionable teens, respond to the desire to look like everybody else. The surgeon's responsibility is to make sure that the teen is looking to refine his or her looks rather than change an identity. Many studies have confirmed that adolescent feelings about identity may change with maturity; thus, refining procedures that could make a person feel better about themselves should never be denied on an ethnic basis. However, if a teen desires procedures that will totally change their identity, motivations need careful evaluation.

Risks

The risks in ethnic surgery, as in any surgery, can be broken down to the physical and the psychological.

Each procedure carries its own physical risks. Many of the operations are standard across cultural lines and are considered mainstream regardless of background. But there are some unique risks inherent to each group. For example, body-contouring surgery and breast surgery involve incisions and therefore scars. People with darker complexions can have darker and thicker scars. If an individual is prone to hypertrophic scars, then introducing them in an attempt to refine a breast is counterproductive and even damaging. Similarly, though nasal surgery can be performed from inside the nose, with hidden incisions, if the patient requires borrowed tissue from elsewhere, the incisions made to obtain the tissue may leave visible scars. The same holds true for the Asian eyelid. In some cases, the scar in the lid, which usually fades into obscurity, can be more obvious. These factors must be evaluated for each patient in the context of the desired procedure.

Aside from the physical challenges, there are psychological risks in performing plastic surgery on teens of any ethnic background, and the surgeon, teen, and parents must make sure the teen is truly ready for surgery. With the exception of breast implants, which can be removed, surgical procedures are permanent; the changes cannot be reversed if the patient changes his or her mind.

Final Thoughts

The hybridization of peoples has created a melting pot of beauty, and concepts of beauty will continue to change. In previous decades, women were more full figured. Now the goal is to be lean. Once, big lips were considered inferior, and surgeons were reducing them, and now surgeons are making them fuller.

On the positive side, patients are rarely running away from their native identity and are most often looking to refine rather than to disguise. On the negative side, many lack understanding of the limitations of some ethnic characteristics. Not all skin types heal the same, and not everyone can have the same magazine result. It is up to the responsible plastic surgeon to say "no" as well as "yes" when the situation warrants it and to provide the patient and family with an overview of the risks as well as the benefits.

13

Cutting Edge or On Thin Ice: Innovations Influencing Teen Plastic Surgery

FINGERTIP FACTS

☞ If it seems too good to be true, it probably is.

☞ Look for procedures that have stood the test of time.

☞ Technology improves surgical skill; it does not replace it.

☞ Think twice before acting once.

EVERYONE LOVES PROGRESS. Patients, friends, and even strangers are always asking me, "What is the latest and greatest in plastic surgery? What is on the cutting edge?" My response is always the same: "If it sounds too good to be true, it is."

We have an expression in plastic surgery: "The enemy of good is great." Simply stated, it means the pursuit of excellence takes time. Great advances are time-tested; that is what makes them great. Many so-called advances are nothing more than media hype playing on the hopes of patients who want quick solutions and are generating expectations that far exceed reality.

Over my thirty-year career, I have seen many procedures based on technologies come and go. One example was a machine that promised to eliminate cellulite. It turned out, for many eager physicians, to be a "$40,000 coatrack," as it failed to deliver any positive results. Every year, new lasers enter the market promising skin-rejuvenating miracles. As soon as the physician obtains one of these lasers—and begins the marathon of expensive lease payments—it becomes obsolete. For a price, the company provides an "upgrade." I have seen "tumescent" liposuction, "ultrasonic" liposuction, "laser" liposuction, "power" liposuction, and finally "smart" liposuction. The only thing smart about it is the company's promoting it to surgeons all too eager to be on the cutting edge. Usually, these doctors who are leaping without looking end up on thin ice!

Microsurgery and Liposuction

Cutting-edge procedures and technologies evolve over time and continue to be refined, and some of them are quite remarkable. Certainly there have been great advances in my field that I am proud to be a part of. Microsurgery and liposuction, for example, have been, in my opinion, two of the greatest leaps we have taken in decades.

Microsurgery has allowed surgeons to transfer tissue from any location in a patient's body to the needed site. What began as an ability to restore amputated parts has evolved into limb and face transplants. Along the way, we learned how to take tissue and make breasts for those devastated by mastectomy.

> Microsurgery has allowed surgeons to transfer tissue from any location in a patient's body to the needed site. What began as an ability to restore amputated parts has evolved into limb and face transplants.

We can reroute nerves to reanimate faces stricken by nerve injury or other facial palsies. We can take parts of bone and replace other bones lost to trauma or disease.

Liposuction redefined a way of thinking in plastic surgery. Before its advent, few would have believed that through a small poke-hole incision, large volumes of fat could successfully be removed to recontour a body. The common thinking at the time was that fat could only be removed as a block of tissue with its attached skin, like in a tummy tuck. Now liposuction is the most common plastic surgical procedure.

> Liposuction redefined a way of thinking in plastic surgery. Before its advent, few would have believed that through a small poke-hole incision, large volumes of fat could successfully be removed to recontour a body.

Microsurgery and liposuction are both the children of new, sophisticated technology. In fact, you could say that what brings a connection to these two very different advances is that they ushered in the era of medical technology. The microscopic device remains constant, but its applications change, allowing for surgical advances. With liposuction, the application remains constant, but the instrumentation keeps changing. Microsurgery is driven by science, whereas liposuction is driven by entrepreneurial changes in the tool itself.

In this chapter, we look at many new "advances" in plastic surgery and apply them to teenage plastic surgical scenarios. Some are truly cutting edge, and some are traps waiting to put patients and surgeons on thin ice.

The Internet

The Internet is probably the world's most far-reaching advance in communication, and it has had both a positive and a negative impact on plastic surgery. On the positive side, it allows for rapid communication between specialists and almost instant access to valuable medical information. Hardly a physician in practice today could function without use of the Internet.

The downside to the Internet is the development of Web marketing and the easy access to incorrect information. These problems affect today's teens in particular because their generation is the most Internet savvy. Teens can surf the World Wide Web and acquire volumes of unfiltered and unedited information posted by individuals who have no authority on the topic. Teens can obtain false information on plastic surgery procedures performed on celebrities and use this information to nurture their own hopes. They are extremely impressionable and could be easily influenced by an ad that doesn't present all the information. In addition to searching sites and reading blogs, they can even set up online consultations using computer cameras. This is usually all done in secret, without parental knowledge, much less consent. Even parents may be misled by the advertorial nature of the information on some Web sites and make poor decisions for their teenagers.

In my practice, I have experienced both the good and the bad from the Internet. On the positive side, it helped me get back in touch with a former patient. A girl I operated on as a baby for a cleft lip and palate moved away shortly after the surgery. Twenty years later, she found me on Facebook. We were able to catch up on each other's lives, and I was able to see how she grew into a beautiful and well-adjusted young woman. Upon her recent graduation from college, she came to see me for a long overdue follow-up. On the negative side, teens visit the office with reams of online articles full of misinformation. Families believe the information to be gospel, and surgeons find themselves on the defensive, trying to bring sanity and reason to a consultation.

The bottom line is that information from the Web, like any other information, must be read critically. Don't take what you read there as divine truth, no matter what site it comes from.

Interlopers

Plastic surgery has exploded in recent years. It is no longer reserved for the very rich, nor is it a hidden practice. Now it is much more affordable, making it accessible to people of any age, gender, race, and background who can pay for it.

As the last bastion of the free-market system in medicine, the field of plastic surgery has drawn many non–plastic surgeon physicians who have been economically damaged by managed care. Severe cuts in re-imbursements have driven these interlopers to dabble in cosmetic med-icine. They obtain weekend certificates and use elaborate advertising touting cutting-edge technologies such as lasers and liposuction tools to lure the unsophisticated researcher into dangerous waters. There are ophthal-mologists, dermatologists, otolaryngologists, gyne-cologists, and internists promoting themselves as cosmetic surgeons. I have even seen a gastroenter-ologist running a liposuc-tion center. His lack of experience resulted in a patient losing a leg from complications. This is a buyer-beware age we are living in—think twice before acting once!

> Plastic surgeons cringe when we see wannabes citing certificates from bogus boards or make-believe societies. I have seen a gastroenterologist running a liposuction center. His lack of experience resulted in a patient losing a leg from complications.

As mentioned in a previous chapter, almost any physician can call himself a "plastic surgeon." Even the term "board certified" can be mis-leading. Board certified in what? A doctor can be certified in a complete-ly different specialty but mislead the prospective patient into linking the certification with plastic surgery. Plastic surgeons, such as myself, who have completed decades of dedicated training cringe when we see wan-nabes citing certificates from bogus boards or make-believe societies. **Remember: It is critical to make sure your plastic surgeon is certified by the American Board of Plastic Surgery—the only board recognized by the American Board of Medical Specialties.**

Medical Spas

Entrepreneurship has seized an opportunity in cosmetic medicine with the medical spa. Once upon a time, you went to a spa to be reinvigo-rated; now there is a belief you can be rejuvenated. Many of these medi-spas advertise physician supervision as technicians inject Botox and fillers into the face and laser the skin to remove unwanted hair and wrinkles. Your teen's facial can turn harmful if you haven't done your research. These spas tout their use of cutting-edge technologies, but these technologies in inappropriate hands can turn eager clients into unhappy patients seeking remedy to problems the spa created.

Many believe that if they are being treated in a spa, the procedure is not dangerous. Their fear of physicians motivates them to go to a medi-spa. Ironically, many of them end up in a physician's office after a medi-spa treatment has caused an infection, a filler has turned into an unwanted lump, or a laser has caused a burn or hyperpigmentation or other damage from trying to bleach and blend irregular pigmentations. I have even removed materials that a medi-spa technician had injected into the wrong places. The patient's lack of knowledge about the spa's expertise resulted in more time, money, and frustration for correction.

If you are looking into medi-spas, get several unbiased referrals on the spa you are considering. Call your local branch of the Better Business Bureau to see if complaints have been lodged, and look at second-party Web sites for comments on the spa's services. Again, don't take any information on faith. Do diligent research, and question everything you are told. Your teen's health and appearance are not to be put in the hands of amateurs.

Ask if your plastic surgeon or dermatologist has a licensed medical aesthetician working in his office. That will insure that these extended spa services are medically supervised.

Tissue Expanders

Tissue expansion has proven to be a truly cutting-edge technique with excellent benefits. Many adults are familiar with its application in breast reconstruction after mastectomy to help create a new pocket for an implant. In the pediatric plastic surgery world, it has revolutionized the way we can remove large nevi, vascular lesions, and burn scars and reconstruct the defects with normal skin. By inserting a tissue expander, or deflated balloon, next to the area to be removed and slowly inflating the balloon (over weeks to months), we can make the skin expand (just as pregnancy slowly expands the abdomen). When the lesion is removed, the expanded skin can be slid into place to provide a more natural-looking reconstruction than the unsightly skin grafts of the past. Tissue expanders come in all sizes and can even be custom made if needed.

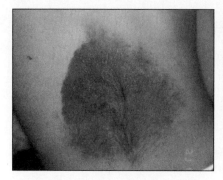

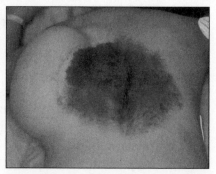

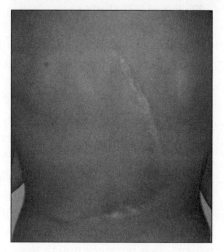

Large congenital hairy nevus on the back on a 3-year-old girl. Tissue expansion of the adjacent skin will allow for complete removal and reconstruction. An acceptable scar seen fifteen years later. The skin post-surgery and recovery is soft and like the rest of her back. Before the advent of tissue expansion, a large and unsightly skin graft would have been needed.

Some of my best reconstructions in children were made possible with tissue expansion. I had a child patient with a significant burn scar on her scalp. A large portion of her hair was missing. By placing a tissue expander under a part of her scalp with hair and slowly inflating it, I was able to provide healthy, hairy scalp to cover the bald area. Similarly, I was able to remove a giant, hairy nevus occupying one-fourth of the front of another patient's scalp and replace it with healthy scalp and hair. Gone was the potentially malignant tissue and in its place normal scalp.

In the capable hands of a real plastic surgeon, tissue expansion is on the positive side of cutting edge—an advancement that has allowed complex skin problems to find successful solutions.

Fat Grafting

Cutting-edge science has shown two things about fat: one, it harbors stem cells; and two, when it's transferred, fat takes on the feel of adjacent tissue.

The first fact presents the exciting possibility that fat could lessen the demand for embryonic stem cells. In the future, patients in need of stem cells for treatment of disease or to regenerate damaged organs might be able to obtain them from liposuction aspirate—fat siphoned off by a liposuction procedure.

The second fact, as mentioned earlier in the book, means that we can transfer fat to structurally change a face or body. When I work on bringing facial balance to teens I have found fat grafting extremely useful. It allows me to augment teens' chins and cheeks as well as fill small defects with living tissue. It is easy to obtain the small amounts of fat needed to effect a change, and the recovery is rapid and almost painless. More than 50 percent of the transferred fat is present five years later.

Clinical research is ongoing to see if this technique could work as an alternative to silicone implants for augmenting small breasts. This technique could possibly fill a need for older teens psychologically suffering from lack of breast development. At this writing, enhancement is limited to one cup size. When large volumes of fat are required, the patient must be large enough to be a source for the fat. The risk of infection is low with small fat transfers but increases with the larger grafts. In addition, fat can sometimes calcify, and those calcifications could be misinterpreted for malignancy in a breast mammogram. Thus, more research is needed.

I have no experience with large-volume fat grafting as would be needed for breasts and buttocks. I am personally too cautious to be the "first on the block" with anything, but I anxiously await new data to allow me to consider this aspect of fat grafting a great advancement as well.

Implants

When most people think of an implant, they think of a breast implant made of silicone. However, implant technology has expanded far beyond silicone breast implants and has many cutting-edge applications.

Facial implants are used all over the facial skeleton in what is called onlay surgery. The surgeon fixes a custom-shaped bone-like implant into the adjacent bone with screws and plates and creates a new three-dimensional shape. Before the surgery, computer programs help the patient and surgeon visualize the new form to be created.

Fillers such as Juvéderm, Radiesse, and Sculptra are common in the world of rejuvenation procedures for adults. Under certain circumstances, these fillers can have beneficial applications for teens. If a patient has an irregularity after a rhinoplasty, a small amount of filler can camouflage the defect, buying time to settle the anxious teen until revisional surgery can be performed. If a patient experiences some nerve weakness after facial surgery, Botox can be used to balance the face until the swelling subsides and nerve function returns. Teens should not use fillers and Botox as adults do. It is expensive, and young faces do not need big lips and lines of facial expression reduced to a flat affect.

Wherever there is a body part, there is a potential place for an implant. As mentioned in a previous chapter, I have negative opinions regarding teen males who get chest implants and teens of both sexes who get calf and buttock implants. It is only a matter of time before a problem arises and the implants need removal. Some may consider this cutting edge but I place them on thin ice. A better solution in the future may be fat grafting.

Lasers

There are books all about laser procedures alone, and there are many different lasers for many different needs. There are lasers that can cut and coagulate, and there are lasers that attack pigments. These lasers can help to remove vascular lesions and many tattoo pigments. Laser technology is always changing, and this can be a good and bad thing.

There are two problems with laser therapies. Lasers can be rented along with a technician. Some surgeons want to use them but lack experience and rely on the technician. If complications arise, these inexperienced surgeons (or non-surgeons dabbling in cosmetics) have no knowledge on how to treat the problem. Then the physician blames the technician, and the technician blames the physician, and they both blame the rental company. The lawyers, on the other hand, have a field day, as the patient proceeds with litigation for the botched procedure.

Other times, because of the expense of the laser, a surgeon may feel compelled to use it when it is not really needed. For example, a doctor may push every patient to have a laser peel to refresh and tighten their skin, regardless of the initial reason for consultation. So do not assume that because your surgeon recommends laser therapies, it is the best way to go.

Tattoo Removal

Tattoos can be very difficult to remove when they're no longer desired. But few teens seeking tattoos envision themselves old and in a nursing home with a wrinkled and faded tattoo, and they can't imagine their tattoos being harmful to a future profession or relationship. I once removed a giant tattoo from a former Hells Angel before the motorcyclist went to nursing school.

As described in chapter 11, once upon a time, surgeons had to cut out tattoos to remove them, which left a residual scar. To some patients, the scar was more explainable ("I was in an accident") than the tattoo. The other option was dermabrading (sanding down the skin) and rubbing salt solutions into the raw wounds to try and leach out pigments. This was time-consuming and yielded only limited results.

Today, we use lasers to remove body art. Each laser frequency has a color that attacks another color. Although time-consuming and much more expensive than the tattoo itself, laser therapy can diminish most tattoos.

The newest cutting-edge technology is tattoo ink that can easily be removed with lasers. Freedom2 Infinitink is the first step toward semi-permanent tattooing (see chapter 11).

Although tattoo removal through lasers and the new removable ink has come a long way, the process is not perfected. Do not sanction tattoos on teens, thinking that they can be painlessly and thoroughly removed. These advances may not happen for many years to come.

Genital Surgery

The most common plastic surgery for genitalia involves surgery for the female labia majora—the outer "lips" of the vagina. Because of the increasing popularity of the Brazilian wax (which removes all pubic hair), this area has become more visible in sexually intimate situations. Labiaplasty can reduce the size of the labia majora to a more comfortable and aesthetically pleasing form. It does not affect any function and is not a circumcision. This procedure is gaining acceptance, and I have received phone calls from mothers inquiring about it for their teen daughters.

> Today, we use lasers to remove body art. Each laser frequency has a color that attacks another color. Although time-consuming and much more expensive than the tattoo itself, laser therapy can diminish most tattoos.

The procedure is quick and can be performed under local anesthesia or light sedation. The recovery is rapid and painless, and activities are limited only by the early swelling. All the stitches absorb on their own, and patients feel back to normal within a week. But as with all such surgeries, this is not something to do unless there is a real issue of embarrassment or physical limitation. The surgery is becoming increasingly popular, however, as teens have become sexually active at younger ages.

Gender Surgery

Transgender surgery (also called sexual-reassignment surgery) is complex and involves many disciplines—plastic surgery, urology, psychiatry, and endocrinology. It should never be taken lightly, because the results are permanent. Research indicates that some young individuals are psychosocially burdened by living in what they perceive as the wrong body for them and that a change earlier rather than later can greatly improve their lives. This research is very new as it relates to teens, and parents considering transgender surgery for their teen should consult only physician teams experienced in gender reassignment. An organization that may help individuals seeking advice in this area is World Professional Association for Transgender Health, Inc. (www.wpath.org), formerly called the Harry Benjamin International Gender Dysphoria Association.

Permanent Makeup

Imbedding ink for eyebrows, eyeliners, and lip colors is no different from other tattooing. The results are permanent. Teens should not consider these procedures because they have yet to experience the effects of aging. Once skin loosens and sags, the permanent makeup will be out of position and cannot be removed.

Final Thoughts

The past fifty years have seen a rapid progression in technology, making surgery better for the patient and the surgeon. We have better lighting, better suture material, better anesthesia, and better instrumentation. For example, the development of endoscopes has allowed surgeons to operate without big incisions and yet see the surgery on the "big screen."

The next decades should be even more exciting. We have begun the journey into fetal surgery to correct birth defects even before the child is born. We have seen transplantation evolve beyond organs like heart and kidneys to the face and limbs. Once we solve the problem of immunologic rejection, there are no limits to what we can accomplish to help amputees and burn and trauma victims.

Researchers are now able to grow skin from small fragments. This cutting-edge technology has been lifesaving for some burn victims. With further research, it seems inevitable that we will eventually be able to grow body parts for transplantation.

When I started practice almost thirty years ago, I had a camera and a pager. Now we have cell phones, BlackBerry devices, electronic records, and computer imaging. We are totally and instantly connected. Computers will only get better, and so will the ability to image and plan patient surgeries. Needles and threads became smaller with the use of the microscope. With the advent of robotics, the surgeons of tomorrow will able to operate a robot remotely and move it into tiny spaces to do the unimaginable.

Plastic surgery has always been on the cutting edge. Whether it's burn research or the study of wound healing or aging, plastic surgeons have been on the forefront. It was a plastic surgeon, Dr. Joseph Murray, who performed the first kidney transplant; he received the Nobel Prize in science. It's unfortunate that media-generated sensationalism has caused a negative public view of plastic surgery. It's hard for people to think of the field in a positive way when they identify it with the treatments chosen by Michael Jackson or Joan Rivers or Pamela Anderson—the ice breaks and the public suffers when information is learned through the tabloids. We can hope, though, that as we achieve even more advances in technology and procedures and more patients benefit from plastic surgery, that the public's opinion of the practice of plastic surgery will also change for the better.

It is hard for any surgeon to counsel a patient on waiting for technology to get better, especially when the physical or emotional need is there. While the ways of doing things will get better in time, we cannot delay the present for a hope in the future. All elective surgery is done at a point in time when the most current and advanced procedures, information, and technologies are used. We live in this day and rely on today.

That being said, there are situations such as balding where surgery in a teen is never the answer. The future is in the genetic research to stop it from happening. We hope that genetic research will also unlock the secrets to preventing obesity, making body contouring an obsolete specialty.

Although technical procedures will become more and more advanced in the coming years, the need for good old-fashioned parenting doesn't change. When considering advanced or more traditional plastic surgical procedures for your teen, add a strong dosage of parental supervision, advice, support, and insight, and you have a winning prescription for your child.

PART THREE

POSTSURGERY

14

Happy Endings
and Beautiful Beginnings

YOU AND YOUR TEEN thought about a plastic surgery procedure, researched it, and finally made the decision to go forward.
Hopefully, all the preparation led you make correct choices. Now
comes that period of adjustment to the physical change from the surgery and the emotions surrounding it.

In this chapter, I talk about what happens outside, as well as inside,
when teens begin the healing and integration process. They have new
bodies; now they must bring this new physical reality into their every-
day life and become comfortable "in their new skin." This is usually a
happy time, but there can be challenges.

Recovery

The recovery room is usually where the patient first begins the integration process. Comments like "I can't believe I did it" are common when
the patient first wakes up with a new body or face.

Most of the cosmetic quality-of-life procedures discussed in this book
are performed ambulatory, meaning that within hours after the operation, the patient will leave the security of the surgical facility and all its

attendant staff to go home. Most surgical facilities require that the patients meet certain criteria before they can be discharged. As a rule, the patient should have fully recovered from anesthesia and be free of any nausea and vomiting. They should have ambulated (gotten up and walked), gone to the bathroom to urinate, and tolerated some liquids by mouth. Once these milestones are met and the surgeon is comfortable that all bandages are clean and intact and that he has the patient's contact information—all of which happens fairly soon after the procedure—the patient is ready to go home. Though most will be happy to be in their own bed, some will experience anxiety. The surgeon's careful preoperative explanations of the entire recovery process go a long way to allay fears for both patient and parent. It is important for the surgeon to understand his patient and for the patient and family to understand the surgeon's postoperative routine.

Parents, ask yourself:

- *Am I calm or anxious in general?* Can I handle the responsibility of my child and the recovery needs? Can I convey information about my child's recovery process over the phone to the doctor when asked?
- *Am I comfortable with an outpatient procedure?* Am I comfortable being the recovery caregiver? Do I need assistance from outside sources—family, friends, or professional visiting nurses? Who will change bandages if needed? Who will help my child to the bathroom? Who will prepare the meals? Who will take him or her to the follow-up appointments?
- *Do I understand the surgeon's postoperative routine?* Am I clear on all the home care instructions such as those on washing, bathing, and showering?
- *Do I know when the follow-up appointments are?*

Ask your teen:

- *Can you comply with the restrictions placed on you as you go through the recovery process?*
- *Have you truly allowed enough time to recover?* Does your school know you will be absent? Do they know you may have physical limitations and restrictions when you return?

Preoperative anxiety and jitters dissipate as the period of recovery begins but reality sets in as the patient must now comply with all of the surgeon's instructions. The first instruction, in my practice, after any procedure is to rest at home. One of the hardest concepts to relate to teenagers is allowing time for healing. If the operation went well and there is little or no pain, teens feel that this is a signal to be out and about—after all, it was just plastic surgery! Teens and their parents must be clear that all plastic surgery is still real surgery, and things can go wrong. The postoperative period is when wounds heal. The patient's cooperation during this time can affect the outcome. There certainly have been cases in all plastic surgery practices in which a lack of compliance on a patient's part changed the results even though the surgery itself was done correctly.

Different operations require different recovery periods, and different surgeons have different routines they want the patient to follow. Doctor–patient relationships can suffer if the family doesn't acknowledge and comply with the routines. I have encountered anger from teen patients because they interpreted feeling good as a signal to be out with their friends during early recovery. My strong advice against that was interpreted as too controlling. Teens often live in the moment and do not see the long view. A parent's role is to act as the surgeon's advocate during the recovery period. This is critical to your child's recovery.

Unveiling

When discharged, patients are often in bandages or splints. This means that they can't yet see their results; they can only imagine them. The first dressing change is often anxiety-provoking to the patient and family, as this is when the results are unveiled. The patient will have postoperative swelling and bruising, something everyone should be briefed on beforehand. Some first dressing changes include removal of drains. Although not painful, the removal is certainly unfamiliar to most, and it can be startling to witness a long tube emerging from the surgical site. Sometimes the patient is calm, but family members in the room get faint or translate their anxiety to the teen. Parents should make every effort to remain calm during the dressing change for their teen's sake.

219

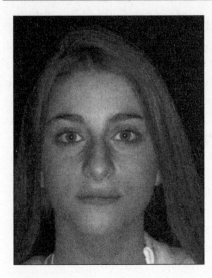

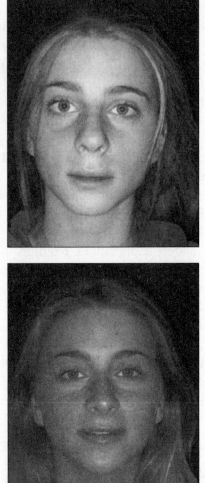

The final result is not always what is seen when the bandages come off. There is often swelling and bruising. The patient needs support through this transition period while waiting for their final result. The first shows pre-op nasal deformity, the second depicts swelling and bruising immediately after cast removal, and the third is the girl six months after surgery with the refined final result.

Seeing fresh incisions for the first time can also be disturbing, and the patient may feel many emotions. Some are immediately ecstatic, some are tentative, and some are even disappointed because they were hoping for instant healing and an immediate final result. Compassion and understanding on the part of the surgeon and office staff is critical; the adolescent is in uncharted waters, and the family is likely to respond to the emotions of the child. Your surgeon should reassure your teenager that what they are seeing is what he expected. Many patients are relieved when they are rebandaged and covered back up. It is usually at this point, when they see how fresh and new the incisions are, that teens understand the need for compliance in recovery.

> Dear Dr. Lukash,
> Thank you so much for the care you gave our daughter. This was a very frightening procedure for us as parents, but you allayed our fears as much as possible. You kept us fully informed of what to expect and how you would proceed. You and your entire staff provided an atmosphere of clinical expertise and professionalism combined with warmth and caring. I cannot imagine our daughter in more capable hands.
> —P & K G. (parents)

Facial Surgery

When a nasal splint is removed, patients often need to catch their breath before looking at their results. If there is swelling, the surgeon should explain it before they look, so they understand that this is not their final result. Even when the surgery has gone exactly as planned, some teens are not prepared for the change. The reflection in the mirror is no longer familiar, and they may need a period of hand-holding as they adjust.

The nose is frequently tender, and teens can be squeamish about touching it or cleaning their nostrils. They may be reluctant to perform any massage maneuvers to reduce swelling for fear of pain and disturbing the result. Gentle encouragement from the surgeon and family goes a long way. I frequently show my patients and their parents how to tape the nose at night to reduce swelling after the splint has been removed. They remove the tape each morning before school. This proactive involvement with their new nose helps them in their transition. In addition, the nose often feels numb and therefore foreign to their face. The teen should be warned about potential sunburns.

If the patient has also had a chin or cheek augmentation, he or she may need more adjustment time. In spite of office staff admiration and family support, the teen may still be anxious about the change. If the result is slow to appear because of excess bruising, the teen may feel more disappointment than happiness. Only time and support will get him through the transitional period to new normalcy. To help a teen at this point in recovery, I review the initial computer-imaged plan and then show examples of other patients at that stage. This lets him know his is on course and will realize our hoped-for results.

Skin Surgery

Every incision leaves its mark, and even though the mole has been removed and the remaining scar is small, it is different from what the patient was used to. The teen may at first focus more on what is left than the original problem. Time will be needed to adjust. Proactive interventions such as massage and topical creams may help in allaying anxiety during healing.

Ear Surgery

Ears can swell and bruise, but when the bandages come off at one week, most kids are immediately pleased with their results. However, they still need to take it easy. It is vital that as a parent you support your doctor's insistence that your child not do too much too soon. You don't want him or her to undo the result before the ears have had time to heal. I ask my patients to wear a headband over their ears for another three to four weeks for additional protection. Girls with long hair are usually compliant; boys often give parents, and me, a hard time.

Breast and Body Surgery

Breasts are frequently swollen and bruised after surgery. It takes time for the tissues to settle down. Oftentimes, the breasts will seem uneven at first. A breast-reduction surgery on a male may not even appear to have been done at first glance because of swelling. Time is the best friend of healing. The same goes for body-contouring surgeries, such as abdominoplasty. Gravity brings swelling to the bottom of the incision; time and the compression garments take it away.

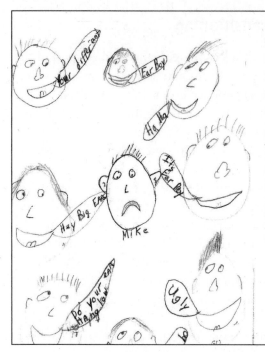

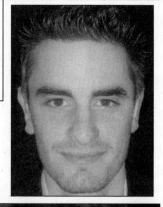

A 9-year-old boy with very prominent ears. His drawing clearly illustrates his despair at being tormented. One year later his face is balanced and his "art" reflects his happiness with his change. The same boy as a young adult."

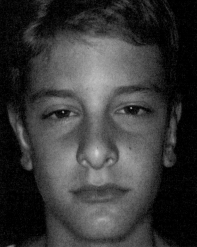

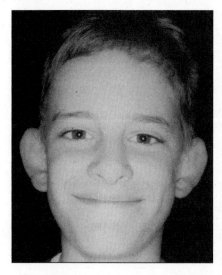

Transitioning

This is the period when the teen needs the guidance and support of the office the most. The incisions are fresh, and scars may appear worse before they begin to fade. The experience is new to the teen *and* the parents, and parents can find it difficult to provide the needed emotional support. It is up to the surgeon to bridge the gap. This is yet another reason it's so important to do research and find a good doctor who is supportive from beginning to end.

Irene's attestation serves as a reminder that emotions and family dynamics can override presurgical explanations. Her teen daughter, who had undergone facial-balancing surgery, was content and in control at every office visit but would lose it when she was with her mother because her mother was not supportive in a positive way and was always probing: "Are you okay?" "Are you sure you are okay?" This situation required daily support phone calls to the anxious mother. When I spoke to the teen, she was always fine.

In my practice, I see patients frequently in the early postoperative period—sometimes twice a week. I then wean them to once a week, then once every two weeks, once a month, once every three months, once every six months, and finally once a year. Letting a teen go too soon can create a sense of abandonment, which will only depress the teen and anger the parents. I never say a final good-bye. I want the teens to feel that they can always communicate with me and that I am there for them. In their rapidly changing world, I try to be a constant.

> Dear Dr. Lukash,
>
> Thank you so much for what you have done for my daughter. She will look absolutely beautiful once the swelling subsides. Sorry for all the neuroses. She was not prepared for the "transitional" phase of cosmetic surgery. I am no better.
>
> —Irene (mother)

Fitting In

As noted throughout this book, teens want to fit in, not make a statement. Adults may use surgery to see a big change—large breasts, flat bellies, lifted faces—to try to rise above the crowd, but teens want to be a part of the crowd. Many adults will openly speak of their surgeries; teens, on the other hand, are quite reticent. Teens like to cope with their metamorphoses quietly by using certain strategies:

1. Timing the surgery during a transition period such as the summer between senior year of high school and freshman year of college— a time after which there is naturally a new beginning.
2. Having surgery over a long vacation when healing can be well under way and the teen has time to adjust.
3. Opting for body surgery in the winter months so that changes can be hidden under clothing.
4. Changing hairstyles to deflect attention to facial surgery.
5. Getting psychological counseling, if needed, to deal with the possible peer response to the change. A teen patient of mine was tormented by his very prominent ears. Surgery to correct them was successful, but he was still emotionally bullied over his surgery. Counseling helped him understand the nature of bullying and gave him strategies to deal with bullies.
6. Seeking dental care, if needed, to brighten and straighten teeth. A new smile could complement a new nose or chin.
7. Changing their wardrobe to help deflect attention from the surgery and to create a new image.

Plastic surgery can be one spoke on the wheel of self-esteem. For the wheel to spin evenly, all the spokes need to be there and be in balance. Surgery alone will not lead to happiness or change a life. It can provide a missing link when all else is in harmony. I hope that this book conveys this message, with all its attendant shades of gray, and does not imply that plastic surgery is the panacea for teen angst. It certainly is not.

Your teen at his or her best is more than just looking good. He or she needs to feel good. Pride in dress and grooming, success in schoolwork, and participation in social activities all contribute to personal bests. We as pediatric plastic surgeons take pride and pleasure in seeing our patients become their best and feel invigorated by those successes. These are our happy endings and your son's and daughter's beautiful beginnings.

Sad Scott to Glad Scott: Years Later

Dear Dr. Lukash,

First off, I hope all is well with you and your family.

I began thinking about you tonight. I was looking through my Facebook account and was trying to find some good pictures to put up. It was then I thought of a picture that would say more about me than any other could. You know as well as I; it is "Sad Scott, Glad Scott." It was at this point I thought about what my life was like back then. And I also think of the way that I am now because of my time with you. You didn't give me a way to hide behind a deformity; you simply gave me a way to feel normal.

See, although I had the surgery very young I never forgot about it through my entire life. Whether it was my first day of junior high, or my first dance in high school, I was able to look at myself proudly. Not because of the fact that I looked normal, but because of the fact that I knew what it was like to be different. My life became easier because of a very simply procedure. Would I have been ashamed of keeping my big elephant ears? No, but did the change boost my self-esteem and make me a stronger person for it? Yes!

Although I am much older now, I still think of the time you gave me. I am working as a chef in Woodstock, Vermont. (It would be an honor if you visited me at the Woodstock Inn. Please take this seriously; it would be great to have you up here for a visit.) But through my culinary career I spent most [of my] time away from the public. But when I do interact with the public I feel more confident because I know I look normal. I could have lived my life with my big ears, but I didn't have to. The fact that I was able to become so comfortable gave me the freedom to be a very open person. I am known as very fun, exotic, loud, understanding, crazy, and—most important of all—a person that other people don't forget.

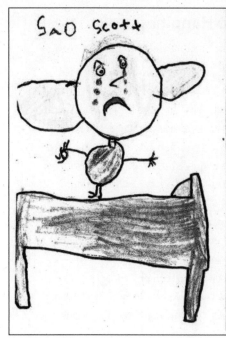
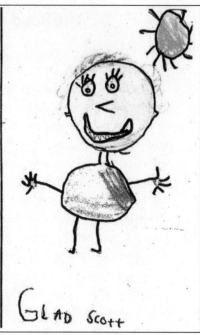

Before surgery Scott draws his perception of how his ears look. He accentuates his unhappiness by drawing tears and telling us he is "sad."

After surgery Scott is happy and draws normal ears. His tears are gone, the sun is out and he is smiling; all clues to his happiness. To punctuate it he tells us he is "glad."

In closing, Dr. Lukash, I hope you know that even years later a small boy still remembers you. And the hero that you became to him. I thank you and thank you a hundred times more. I know through all the years you have given this chance to so many others.

Forever in your debt,

—Scott

The Road to Happiness

Dear Dr. Lukash,

I am writing this letter to let you know how much you have changed my life. In April of 1994 at the age of 15 I was hospitalized for anorexia nervosa. Prior to that I struggled with weight issues, probably related to my early and large breast development. Although my eating was under control by age 16, I continued to struggle with my feelings about my body. I stared at my chest and felt that this represented my entire being.

I have seen many doctors in my life but when I walked into your office I felt a difference. You made me feel calm, assured, and hopeful. From the initial consultation through the breast reduction I felt secure under your care.

Since the surgery I have become a different person. I feel more free and at one with my body. I wear clothes that fit my body instead of large baggy ones to hide my breasts. Thank you for changing my life.

—Laura

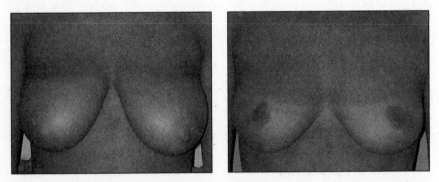

Breast reduction balances her body and provides physical as well as emotional comfort.

The Psychology of Integrating Outward Change
by Dr. Glenn Pollack

Now that surgery is complete and the structural change successful, will it change your teen's feelings about perception by others? No doubt the teen probably feels better regarding the physical change in appearance. However, this does not guarantee that perceptions of how others view them have indeed been altered. These perceptions still might hinder their social confidence, and the teen may continue to suffer from an elevated level of social anxiety. This in turn can continue to inhibit the behavior needed for social assertiveness and affect the ability to acquire and even maintain friendships—the social glue that binds people together in the outside world.

How we interpret situations plays a significant role in determining our behavior. Cognition changes do not always follow surgical changes, and at times, a patient might require another type of professional support: a therapist who can help a child or adolescent reframe or reinterpret how others view him or her. Misinterpretation can make someone prone to social rejection. The child or teen who perceives that he will not know what to say, or thinks that he may act awkwardly in front of his peers or others, needs to be reeducated.

Watch your teen for signs that they may need help reinterpreting social cues and messages. If teens have lived all their lives believing that others do not like them based on appearance, they may have a hard time believing that they are now liked for themselves and not their "new" nose or bodies.

A trained counselor or therapist is invaluable support during this time. Never be ashamed to seek help, even if you feel the process of transformation is completed. A teen may turn from a caterpillar into a butterfly but still see the former. Guidance and caring support will help to develop a new mind-set, new social cues, and new acceptance of self and others.

Afterword

I HOPE THAT AS YOU READ through this guide to teenage plastic surgery you realized how plastic surgery can help a young person at a critical crossroads in life. It is to be used only for the right patient for the right reason at the right time. When that happens, there is no greater joy for a surgeon.

I also want you, as a parent, to realize that there are many sides to plastic surgery—some you may not have thought of or may have viewed with a negative bias. I will consider this book successful if readers take a deep breath and think about the considerable positives that plastic surgery offers rather than the negative press that follows celebrity dalliances and demeans hard-working, moral, and ethical surgeons who are trying to make a beneficial difference in their patients' lives.

My decision to go into aesthetic surgery for teens, and my idea to write this book, were not spontaneous. They evolved over time as I looked closely at the lives of children whose physical conditions were deemed deformities or very much outside the realm of normal. Pediatric plastic surgeons struggle to repair cleft lips and palates and to build ears where there are none. We never give up trying to make children the best they can be.

Quality-of-life surgery is the blending of the reconstructive and the cosmetic. If each child is an individual with his or her own set of anxieties, who should determine where the boundary between reconstruction and cosmetics lies? Is replacing an absent ear reconstructive but repairing an ear that protrudes not? And just how much does it need to project for correction to be acceptable? Is a nasal deformity from a cleft lip worthy of correction but a nose with a large bump not? One child at a time has taught me that each person has his or her own life independent of others, and each child's feelings about how he or she looks need to be taken seriously.

Plastic surgery is not and never will be the magic wand to erase the anxieties surrounding adolescence. It can, however, be an important spoke on that wheel of self-esteem. I hope that all children will be given a fair chance to express how they feel about their appearance. I hope that adults will listen without being too judgmental.

Those of us who have dedicated our lives to plastic surgery are physicians first, and we owe it to our patients to listen to them. Together with parents and other health professionals, we aim to be a response team that can intercede to benefit the growing and developing adolescent.

I leave you with a positive visual of the value of plastic surgery to young lives. The following are a few more of my patients' artistic expressions about appearance and self-esteem.

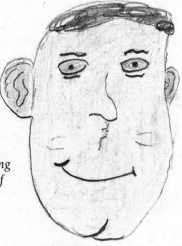

After surgery Sad Jeff from Chapter 1 is smiling and draws a normal self portrait.

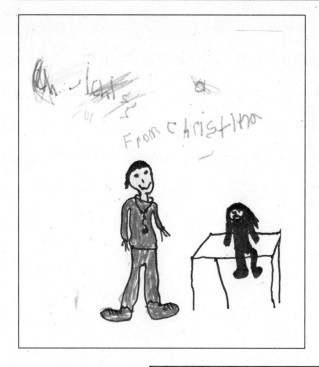

A 10-year-old girl with scar deformities and facial imbalance from a cleft lip and palate. Before revision surgery she places herself in the rear of the picture and is monochromatic, small and dark. She views herself as non-descript. The doctor is large, happy, colorful and in the front of the picture. He represents hope.

After surgery to refine her lip and nose she is colorful and large and the doctor recedes. She has renewed self-esteem. Her drawing demonstrates a willingness to socialize and a diminishing dependence on her doctor.

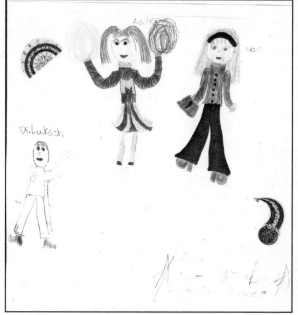

233

Resource Guide

American Society of Plastic Surgeons (ASPS)
Established in 1931, the ASPS is the largest organization of plastic surgeons in the world. All members are certified by the American Board of Plastic Surgery. The Web site is user friendly and has a consumer information section.
www.plasticsurgery.org
847-228-9900
444 E. Algonquin Rd.
Arlington Heights, IL 60005

American Society for Aesthetic Plastic Surgery (ASAPS)
Established in 1967, the ASAPS is an organization of board-certified plastic surgeons specializing in cosmetic surgery. Its mission is both education and patient advocacy.
www.surgery.org
888-272-7711

American Association of Pediatric Plastic Surgeons (AAPPS)
The AAPPS is an organization of plastic surgeons dedicated to plastic surgery for children. It is affiliated with the American Society of Plastic Surgeons and the American Academy of Pediatrics.
www.plasticsurgery.org/About_ASPS/Links_to_Related_Organizations/American_Association_of_Pediatric_Plastic_Surgeons.html
847-434-7668
141 Northwest Point Blvd.
Elk Grove, IL 60007

American Association for Accreditation of Ambulatory Surgery Facilities (AAAASF)

The AAAASF was established in 1980 to ensure the highest standards of safety in ambulatory facilities. More than 1,000 facilities are in compliance. The organization's Web site is very patient friendly and informative.

www.aaaasf.org

888-545-5222

5101 Washington St., Ste. #2F

Gurnee, IL 60031

American Academy of Dermatology (AAD)

The AAD is the main society for dermatologists and maintains a large Web site that addresses many FAQs about skin health and disease.

www.aad.org

866-503-7546

P.O. Box 4014

Schaumburg, IL 60168

American Society for Laser Medicine and Surgery (ASLMS)

The ASLMS is a society dedicated to excellence with regards to biomedical technology as it relates to the use of lasers.

www.aslms.org

715-845-9283

2100 Stewart Ave., Ste. 240

Wausau, WI 54401

American Psychiatric Association (APA)

The APA's educational site answers questions and provides resources for help with psychiatric issues.

www.psych.org

888-357-7924

1000 Wilson Blvd., Ste. 1825

Arlington, VA 22209

American Society for Metabolic and Bariatric Surgery (ASMBS)

Founded in 1983, the ASMBS is dedicated to the improvement of public health and well-being by lessening the burdens of obesity. The site has educational as well as resource information for patients.

www.asmbs.org

352-331-4900

100 SW 75th St., Ste. 201

Gainesville, FL 32607

American Society of Anesthesiologists (ASA)

Founded in 1905, the ASA is dedicated to excellence in anesthesia and pain relief. The Web site will help you understand the significant role of the anesthesiologist as part of the surgical team.

www.asahq.org
847-825-5586
520 N. Northwest Hwy.
Park Ridge, IL 60068

Children's Access to Reconstructive Evaluation and Surgery (CARES) Act

The act is legislation presently before Congress to provide insurability for children with congenital and traumatic deformities.

House of Representatives Resolution 1339
Sponsor: Carolyn McCarthy (D-NY)

Teen-Longitudinal Assessment of Bariatric Surgery (Teen-LABS)

Teen-LABS is an ancillary study of the Longitudinal Assessment of Bariatric Surgery to evaluate efficacy of bariatric surgery in adolescents and teens.

www.niddklabs.org

Works Consulted

Adato, A. 2006. Too Young for Lipo? *People* 66 (20, November 13).

American Psychiatric Association. 2000. *Diagnostic and Statistical Manual of Mental Disorders,* 4th Ed., Text Revision. Washington, DC: American Psychiatric Association.

Banner, L. 1983. *American Beauty.* Chicago: University of Chicago Press.

Blum, V. 2003. *Flesh Wounds: The Culture of Cosmetic Surgery.* Berkeley and Los Angeles: University of California Press.

Cash, T., and T. Pruzinsky, eds. 2004. *Body Image.* New York: The Guilford Press.

Dion, K., and E. Berscheid. 1974. Physical Attractiveness and Peer Perception Among Children. *Sociometry* 37 (1):1–12.

Dunlap, K. 1920. *Personal Beauty and Racial Betterment.* St. Louis: C. V. Mosby Company.

Etcoff, N. 1999. *Survival of the Prettiest: The Science of Beauty.* New York: Doubleday.

Haiken, E. 1997. *Venus Envy: A History of Cosmetic Surgery.* Baltimore: Johns Hopkins University Press.

Jeffes, S. 1998. *Appearance Is Everything: The Hidden Truth Regarding Your Appearance and Appearance Discrimination.* Pittsburgh: Sterling House.

Lukash, F. N. "Children's Art as Helpful Index of Anxiety and Self Esteem with Plastic Surgery." *Journal of Plastic and Reconstructive Surgery,* v 109 n6 May 2002.

Macgregor, F. C. 1974. *Transformation and Identity: The Face and Plastic Surgery.* New York: Quadrangle Press.

Maliniak, J. 1934. *Sculpture in the Living: Rebuilding the Face and Form by Plastic Surgery.* New York: Lancet Press.

McNeill, D. 2000. *The Face.* Boston: Little, Brown and Co.

Ojeda, A., ed. 2002. *Teen Decisions: Body Image.* San Diego: Greenhaven Press.

Sarnoff, D., and J. Swirsky. 1998. *Beauty and the Beam: Your Complete Guide to Cosmetic Laser Surgery.* New York: St. Martin's Griffin.

Wolf, N. 2002. *The Beauty Myth.* New York: Harper Perennial.

Glossary

Abdominoplasty—"Tummy tuck"; procedure in which excess skin of the abdomen is removed and muscles are tightened.

American Society of Plastic Surgeons—Largest organization of board-certified plastic surgeons in the world. Provides educational resources for members and patients.

Body-contouring surgery—Procedures to address the laxity in skin following significant weight loss. These include brachioplasty (arm lift), abdominoplasty (tummy tuck), thigh lift, and mastopexy (breast lift). May be termed "body lift" when these procedures are combined.

Body dysmorphic disorder—A psychological disorder affecting 1 percent of the population in which the sufferer has an extremely exaggerated perception of a perceived physical flaw.

Brachioplasty—"Arm lift"; procedure in which laxity of the upper arm is removed and tightened after weight loss.

Centers of Excellence—Designation given to institutions that offer specialized team approaches to complex medical problems.

Collagen—Proteins that make up the structural building blocks of body tissues. With age, collagen strength and elasticity decreases and structural integrity weakens.

Cosmetic surgery tourism—Surgery performed off American shores that is usually discounted and often tied to vacation packages.

Cryptotia—Congenital deformity of the upper pole of the ear. Part of a complex ranging from prominent ears to absent ears (microtia).

Facial harmony—The aesthetic beauty of a face in mathematical terms. Harmonious facial structures often fit into the balanced proportions of the Golden Mean.

Fat grafting—Transfer of fat cells from one part of the body to another—most often the chin, cheeks, and lips—to augment structure. Also known as liposculpture.

Genioplasty—Surgery on the chin most often with implants or by advancing the bone (sliding genioplasty).

Gynecomastia—Presence of "breasts" in males that may be fatty and/or glandular in composition.

Hypertrophic scars—Incisions or wounds that heal with pronounced, thick scars.

Implants—Surgical products, most commonly made of silicone, used to augment structures such as breasts and chins.

Keloids—Scars from incisions or wounds that overheal and extend beyond the site of injury.

Labiaplasty—A surgical procedure to reduce enlarged vaginal labia.

Lasers—Machines that use specific wavelengths of energy to provide treatments for vascular lesions, tattoo removal, hair removal, and resurfacing of skin for rejuvenation and stimulation of collagen.

Liposuction—Surgical body-contouring technique in which excess fat is removed through small incisions with vacuum-assisted tubes.

Macromastia—Enlarged female breasts. Also known as mammary hypertrophy.

Macrotia—Condition in which ears are larger than the normal.

Mastopexy—Breast lift to rejuvenate sagging breasts by tightening the skin and repositioning the nipples.

Medi-spa—Facility offering nonsurgical rejuvenations including facials, chemical peels, laser therapies, Botox, and filler injections.

Microsurgery—Surgical techniques to unite small nerves and blood vessels to allow for transplantation and reimplantation of tissues and body parts.

Microtia—Congenital absence of an ear.

Nevi—Moles, or beauty marks, which can range from cosmetic distractions to malignancies. Can be located anywhere on the body and should be checked by a dermatologist if a change is noted.

Nipple grafting—Part of a type of breast reduction surgery in which the nipple is removed and replaced into a more youthful position.

Onlay surgery—Surgery that uses implants to augment the facial skeleton, as opposed to cutting and advancing the bones.

Otoplasty—Surgical procedure to correct the prominent-ear deformity in which sutures are used to re-create the normal folds in the ear.

Panniculectomy—Surgical procedure to remove the excess hanging skin of the abdomen (pannus) after significant weight loss.

Pediatric plastic surgery—Subfield of plastic surgery in which patients are children and that involves all the disciplines within the field: craniofacial, hand, microsurgery, and cosmetic.

Quality-of-life surgery—Procedures to improve the self-esteem of the affected individual. Also called life-enhancing surgery.

Relaxed skin tension lines—Creases in the skin that are perpendicular to the muscles beneath and are favorable places for ideal scar formation. Wounds and incisions that fall with in the RSTL heal the best.

Rhinoplasty—Nose surgery (commonly called a "nose job").

Tissue expansion—Techniques to increase the surface area of skin needed for reconstruction usually using deflated implanted surgical "balloons" that, when slowly inflated, expand the tissue.

W- and Z-plasty—Surgical techniques to rearrange scars to bring them as close the relaxed skin tension lines as possible.

About the Author

FREDERICK N. LUKASH, MD, FACS, FAAP, has consistently been voted one of "America's Top Doctors" by the Castle Connolly guide and by the Consumers' Research Council of America (www.consumersresearchcncl. org). A board-certified cosmetic and reconstructive plastic surgeon in practice in New York City and Long Island since 1981, he is an assistant clinical professor of surgery at the Albert Einstein College of Medicine. He is a fellow in the American College of Surgeons and the American Academy of Pediatrics.

Dr. Lukash is a member of all the major plastic surgical societies—the American Society for Aesthetic Plastic Surgery, the American Association of Plastic Surgeons, the American Association of Pediatric Plastic Surgeons, the American Society of Maxillofacial Surgeons, and The American Society of Plastic Surgeons, for which he is the media spokesperson on the topic of teens and plastic surgery. He has also been involved with the Plastic Surgery Research Council, the American Cleft Palate-Craniofacial Association, Operation Smile, and Surgical Aid to Children of the World.

He has written many articles and textbook chapters for the academic plastic surgery community, including a position paper on plastic surgery for teenagers. This is his first book for the general public.

Dr. Lukash received his college and medical degrees from Tulane University. His postgraduate training in surgery and plastic surgery includes Emory University, State University of New York, and Harvard University, where he held the position of Instructor in Surgery.

Consult www.drlukash.com for his complete educational and academic profile and professional accomplishments.